ADVANCES IN PEDIATRIC SPORT SCIENCES

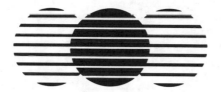

VOLUME ONE
BIOLOGICAL ISSUES

Edited by Richard A. Boileau, Ph.D.

Human Kinetics Publishers, Inc.
Champaign, Illinois

Copy Editor: Peg Goyette
Typesetters: Sandra Meier and Yvonne Sergent
Text Layout: Lezli Harris
Cover Design and Layout: Jack Davis

ISSN: 0748-6375
ISBN: 0-931250-71-4

Printed in the United States of America

10 9 8 7 6 5 4 3 2 1

Human Kinetics Publishers, Inc.
Box 5076   Champaign, IL 61820

Contents

About the Series

Advances in Pediatric Sport Sciences, or APSS, is an interdisciplinary series published every other year. Scholarly reviews pertaining to children and physical activity will be reported in each volume, with Volume 1 and each subsequent odd numbered volume focusing on *biological issues*. Volume 2, and each subsequent even numbered volume, will focus on *behavioral issues*.

Topics covered under biological issues include physiological, biomechanical, medical, and some topics within motor control and development as they pertain to pediatric sport sciences. Behavioral issues will draw upon other topics within motor control and development, sport and exercise psychology, sociology of sport, and anthropology of sport and play.

The series is intended to help advance our understanding of children and their health and well-being as they participate in physical activity. Organized sport, play, and fitness activities are common forms of physical activity that will frequently be considered in the series, but they will not be the only forms considered.

The editor for each volume is selected by the publisher. Persons who may be interested in contributing to the series are encouraged to contact the publisher to learn who the editors are for forthcoming volumes.

Dr. Thomas Gilliam suggested this series to the publisher and was instrumental in organizing the first volume. His contribution is warmly acknowledged.

Preface

Physical activity is perhaps the most commonly observed behavior of children and youth whether in play, exercise, or sport. The activity level of the pediatric population as a whole is increasing. The growing awareness of the health and fitness benefits of exercise among adults is having a positive effect on children and youth. Moreover, despite the apparent decline or lack of growth in school physical education and sports programs, youth appear to be participating in sports and community recreational programs in greater numbers than ever.

The past 50 years have seen substantial growth in our base of knowledge concerning the effect of physical activity on health, fitness, wellbeing, and physical performance. Most of what is known about human physical activity, however, has come from research on adults. Too often, the adult model is simply scaled for size and assumed to fit the child. Although the fallacy of this approach has long been recognized, few researchers today focus on the study of children in physical activity. Consequently our understanding of the interaction of physical activity, growth, development, and maturation is rather limited.

Volume 1 of *Advances in Pediatric Sport Sciences: Biological Issues* is a series of scholarly reviews specifically directed toward the influence of physical activity on children in the context of health, physical performance, and sports medicine issues. Within this general focus, the status of our knowledge is presented concerning the morphological development and cardiorespiratory responses and adaptations of children to physical activity. Additionally, the child's responses to various thermal environments, as well as the influence of physical activity on coronary heart disease risk factors, obesity, diabetes, and orthopedic sports injuries, are examined. In most of these reviews the authors also have addressed the pitfalls of past research and have suggested future research directions within their respective areas.

Sincere appreciation is extended to several individuals who have made this volume possible. First, I am grateful to the participating authors for their contribution and the patience and understanding they have displayed throughout the editorial process. I also thank Debra Bemben, Joy Bunt, Deb Shilts, and Rae Jean Stillman, as well as several unnamed reviewers for assistance in organizing and preparing the manuscripts. Lastly, appreciation is extended to Human Kinetics Publishers for their willingness to support this review series and for their assistance in the editorial and production aspects of this volume.

Richard Boileau

1

Physical Activity and "Wellness" of the Child

Roy J. Shephard
University of Toronto

THE DEFINITION OF "WELLNESS" —
A HISTORICAL PERSPECTIVE

As a laudable objective, "wellness" of the child is second only to motherhood. However, many physicians and parents believe that their potential contribution to this objective has been satisfied if the customary schedule of immunizations is followed and the child develops a pleasing plumpness. The monumental study of "A thousand families in Newcastle Upon Tyne" (136), although subtitled "An approach to the study of health and illness in children," discussed morbidity and mortali-

1

ty rather than health. The U.S. Child Research Council conducted a longitudinal study of healthy growth and development in the Denver area (88), but health records comprised details of the "frequency, duration, severity and type of illnesses and injuries." Even a report on the "health supervision of young children" prepared by the American Public Health Association (6) confined its discussion of attitudes to health to such items as dependence upon the physician, respect for disease-causing agents such as bacteria, sensitivity to emotional disturbances, and acceptance of illness. This limited perspective was particularly unfortunate, considering that the same report stressed that a third to a half of pediatric consultations were for the purpose of health supervision rather than the treatment of illness.

Health remains difficult to define. It is equally difficult to measure. Sorochan (135) spoke of a unity of body, mind, and spirit, a condition wherby an individual could live happily and attain his or her goals. Selye (113) described health as an optimal adaptation of the body's defense mechanisms to the ravages of stress-producing events. Perhaps most widely quoted has been the World Health Organization's definition of health as "a state of complete physical, mental and social well-being and not merely the absence of disease or infirmity" (153).

Reasons for a delayed acceptance of a broad definition of wellness and health are not difficult to understand. At the time of the WHO statement, the infant mortality rate for Newcastle Upon Tyne was 44 per 1,000, 24 of these deaths occurring in the first month after birth (136); moreover, 1,625 illnesses were treated in the 1,000 infants over the year of observation, even after *excluding* such items as mild colds, minor skin sepsis, sticky eyes, and unclassified respiratory illness. However, advances in social conditions, prenatal care, and the eradication of many infectious diseases have now reduced the infant mortality rate in many developed nations to less than 10 per 1,000, with concurrent decreases in the toll of infectious diseases. Thus the time is ripe for the physician to concentrate his/her efforts upon health and the long-term prognosis of the growing child.

A stronger concern for the positive health of the North American child was first stimulated by studies that compared the minimum muscular fitness of children in the United States, Switzerland, Austria, and Italy (72). The U.S. sample fared poorly for both strength and flexibility items of the Kraus-Weber performance test battery, although the majority of test failures among U.S. children were due to a limited forward reach (99). The limited validity of the Kraus-Weber test soon became apparent, and in 1957 the American Alliance for Health, Physical Education and Recreation (AAHPER) applied a more representative battery of performance tests to 8,500 U.S. boys and girls aged 10 to 17 years (55). The anxiety of North American parents was hardly lessened by reports that the U.S. children performed more poorly than British (18), Danish (67), South African (134), and Japanese (93) youth; indeed, the Oriental investigators commented that "the danger was now in Japanese youth losing their fitness by trying to live like American youth" (93).

On the strength of such publications, the late President Dwight Eisenhower was persuaded to found the Youth Fitness Council, and his successor, President John Kennedy, made a personal plea for a minimum of 15 minutes of continuous exercise per day in every U.S. grade school (111). The AAHPER performance test battery was reapplied to large samples of U.S. children during 1963-64 and again in 1975. The 1963-64 scores suggested that performance had improved substantially on six of the seven test items, leading to the conclusion that "boys and girls age 10 to 17, are generally more fit today . . . than they were seven years ago" (56, p.7). However, no further change of score was observed in the 1975 test results, and corresponding alarm was registered (56) — "The new national norms are cause for concern. . . . There has been no significant improvement in the fitness of our youth in the last 10 years." More critical observers have noted the major influence of body size (25), experience (67), practice (116), and environment (140) upon test scores. While gains from 1957 to 1965 could represent a response to fitness programs, they might equally be attributable to earlier maturation of the students, recent practice of the test battery, or more favorable environmental conditions while data were being collected.

The prime Canadian spokesman for an increase of child activity has been Dr. Don Bailey of the University of Saskatchewan. At a national conference on fitness and health, he expressed the view that "For the ordinary Canadian child . . . physical fitness . . . seems to be a decreasing function of age from the time we put him behind a desk in our schools" (9). His opinion was supposedly based upon direct measurements of maximum oxygen intake, expressed per kg of body mass. Yet a critical examination of the published report shows that (a) there is no fundamental reason for his supposition that oxygen transport per unit of body mass should remain constant throughout growth, and (b) in any event his figures for this index of fitness show no large decrement until the boys concerned reached an age of 13 years (121).

We may conclude that, until recently, there has been little interest in the positive health of the child, and evidence on the supposed inadequacy of current activity patterns is far from conclusive. Nevertheless, most scientists would agree that the right to achieve and maintain physical health is a fundamental freedom that must be assured to all children (28). This chapter reviews this precept in the following contexts: (a) optimization of general development, (b) realization of physical and intellectual potential, (c) fostering of a healthy lifestyle, (d) improvement of current health, (e) prevention of disease, and (f) avoidance of injury.

OPTIMIZATION OF GROWTH AND DEVELOPMENT

Remarkably little experimental evidence concerns the impact of physical activity upon the general development of the child. Although participants in most sports have a characteristic body build (116,141), this is largely a consequence of initial selection rather than a response to the training that has been undertaken (127).

Animal experiments suggest that optimal growth is encouraged by spontaneous exercise rather than the extremes of caging or enforced activity (46,105). Although the quantity of work performed in many animal training experiments has relevance to the endurance athlete, it is much greater than would be anticipated during the recreation or required physical education of a typical child. Some reports have described slow growth among participants in vigorous sports (112) and other forms of strenuous activity, with a retardation of bone development (65) and a delay of menarche (40). On the other hand, the course of growth was apparently normal in 30 Swedish girls who had become national swimming champions (8). And one group of Negro women who had undertaken strenuous manual labor as children were taller and heavier than control subjects who had not performed physical work during the period of their development (4). Many authors have been content to make cross-sectional comparisons between athletes and the general population, leaving their conclusions open to the objection that the athletes were initially selected for a particular sport on the basis of an abnormal pattern of growth or maturation. Studies of the age of menarche in female athletes have also failed to exclude the possibility that the late appearance of menstruation was due to the excitement of competition (27) or a negative energy balance (39) rather than physical activity per se.

Controlled longitudinal studies are few in number and generally involve small samples (34). Moreover, the subjects concerned were only followed for a short period, so that even if function did increase it remained unclear whether the timing of the growth spurt had changed or the ultimate status of the individual had been improved by the exercise treatment.

The Trois-Rivières regional experiment (128) involved 546 normal primary school students from the Province of Quebec. Entire classes followed either the normal ("control") program (one 40-minute period of physical activity per week, taught by a nonspecialist), or a special program (5 hours per week of required physical education taught by a physical educator). Participants were followed longitudinally throughout the period of their primary education (ages 6 to 12 years). Throughout this time span the principal body dimensions such as height and arm span remained remarkably similar in experimental and control groups. Radiographs of the wrist suggested that maturation of experimental subjects was retarded by an average of 3.6 months relative to controls. This was judged to be a local mechanical response to the increased physical activity, however, since the maturation of the teeth and mandible was accelerated by 1.5 months in the experimental group. It can be argued that a larger effect upon growth might have been observed if (a) observations had continued into the adolescent growth spurt, or (b) the experimental group had been required to undertake the very vigorous training patterns required of some young athletes.

REALIZATION OF PHYSICAL AND INTELLECTUAL POTENTIAL

Physical Potential

It is widely accepted that the sedentary adult operates at less than his or her physical potential. An appropriate training program can increase the ability of the heart and lungs to transport oxygen by at least 20%, while even greater gains of physical performance can be induced (114). Some authors have argued that the adolescent growth spurt, with its characteristic hormonal activity, is a particularly fruitful time to stimulate a training response (7,30). Others have maintained that the young child naturally sustains a high level of habitual physical activity, so that a full realization of physical potential is assured even in the absence of structured physical education.

Cross-sectional comparisons between athletic and sedentary students are marred by uncertainties about the relative contributions of constitution (selection) and training to athletic ability (116). Some authors have attempted to infer trainability by comparing the discrepancy of aerobic power between athletic and sedentary children and adults. However, this approach ignores differences in the intensity of athletic selection at different ages (76); for example, we have observed a progressive recruitment of large and heavily muscled boys to ice hockey teams during the teen years.

Some longitudinal studies have shown substantial gains of maximum oxygen intake (17,30,124), physical working capacity (45), or physical performance (36,38,60,152) when children have been trained, but other investigators have found no response. The negative findings could be explained by an inadequate frequency or duration of training sessions (10), failure to make good use of class time (145), neglect of seasonal variations in fitness (125), and the recruitment of subjects who already had a high baseline level of physical activity or fitness (23,138). There may also be a minimum age at which a program becomes physiologically effective. In the Trois-Rivières experiment, for example, the subjects first showed gains of aerobic power and muscle force relative to controls at 8 years of age (124).

Ekblöm exercised boys between the ages of 11 and 13 years (32). His study suggests that enhanced activity increases not only functional variables such as maximum oxygen intake and muscle force but also dimensional factors such as vital capacity and heart volume. However, a longer observation period would be needed to exclude the possibility that activity had merely speeded the maturation of lung and heart volumes rather than increasing the ultimate size of these organs.

The contribution of physical development to the wellness of the child is more problematical. Many children reduce their daily activity once physical education is no longer required at school (57). Any gains of aerobic power are dissipated a few weeks after training has ceased, although there is some evidence that cardiac hypertrophy may persist for a longer period (8). In an acute sense, the fit child has a superior physical performance and a resultant gain of social status (10), which has a beneficial influence upon body image and intellectual and emotional development (48). The pattern of activity needed to sustain maximum oxygen intake may also have a more long-term value in the prevention of atherosclerotic cardiovascular disease (114). However, the advantage to being left with an enlarged heart is less certain, particularly if aerobic power is curtailed by a cessation of training (92). Some (53), but not all (110), authors have found that in middle-age the enlarged heart of a formerly well trained individual has an increased vulnerability to myocardial ischaemia during a standard exercise test.

The other important question yet to be answered is whether a young child's failure to maximize physical potential imposes a permanent restriction upon his or her response to physical training. The cradle snatchers of the international coaching fraternity plainly believe this is so, although the limited physiological data from an earlier era suggests that the aerobic power of top performers who trained 1 to 2 hours per day was very similar to that now seen in students who have trained for 6 to 8 hours per day since the age of 10 or 11 years. Any advantage of performance that is gained from prolonged training schedules probably is due to skill perfection rather than greater physical potential. Observations on Master's competitors and post-coronary patients show that middle-aged men who have not previously engaged in vigorous physical activity can (if they so wish) train to the point of inducing a 70-80% increase of aerobic power (120). While it is conceivable that even larger gains might have been possible if vigorous activity had been initiated in childhood, it is also difficult to argue that the potential of the average adult is curtailed sufficiently to constitute a loss of wellness.

Intellectual Potential

There are many reports concerning the influence of sports participation or additional physical activity upon the intellectual development of the child. However, strong proof of benefit is lacking (20). Limitations of such investigations include:

• the use of cross-sectional or retrospective data (relating observed academic performance to measures of activity or physical ability) (47);

• studies of special populations such as the mentally handicapped or athletes (48,85), with resultant problems of self-selection;

• halo effects, with teachers rewarding star performers by higher marks (48);

• gains of self-image, because of praise from teachers and peers, that lead to true gains of academic achievement (48);

• the short duration of experimental programs of increased activity; and

• possible side-effects from the curtailment of academic instruction.

Nevertheless, the last few years have seen an increasing interest in body movement as a tool for the academic education or re-education of young children (83). Particular interest was aroused by a report from Vanves that an elementary school program comprising 19.5 hours of intellectual activity and 17.5 hours of physical activity per week led to favorable scores when the pupils took the secondary school entrance examination. However, this study and subsequent projects in Regina and Victoria (84) were observational in type, with obvious dangers of misinterpretation due to a Hawthorne response (151). More recently, the Trois-Rivières regional experiment has provided a controlled prospective trial showing the contribution of added physical activity to the academic achievement of students throughout their years in primary school (149). Gains were statistically significant in grades 2, 3, 5 and 6, with the active students receiving higher marks for French, mathematics, English, and science despite a 13% reduction in academic instruction time.

One difficulty in interpreting such findings is that the marks for primary school students are usually assigned by the classroom teachers. In the Trois-Rivières experiment, 80% of the teachers favored the experimental program and the remaining 20% were neutral rather than opposed to the study. It is thus conceivable that a halo effect may have enhanced scores for classes that were undergoing the additional physical activity. Nevertheless, the advantage of sixth-grade students was at least partially confirmed when they participated in uniform, province-wide examinations. Certainly the results seem sufficient to dismiss one common objection to providing additional instruction in physical education — "lack of curricular time."

Many explanations could be given for why added physical activity may have improved academic marks: The shortened class time may have allowed teachers a fresher and better prepared approach to their students; the activity may have had an immediate arousing effect upon the students, improving their attention to academic instruction; the parents may have given additional coaching at home to compensate for missing lessons. However, the most intriguing possibility is that activity stimulated psychomotor development and thus the cognitive process (100). While such a linkage has been vigorously advocated by Piaget and his colleagues, one must admit that psychomotor function can develop normally despite quite severe mental retardation and that the reverse is also possible (143). In support of the Piaget hypothesis, students participating in the Trois-Rivières study (150) demonstrated (a) an improved perception of body dimensions, (b) a better appreciation of the vertical, and (c) more accurate finger recognition. The advantage of the active students was greatest during the first 2 years of school, with control students making up for much of their deficiency as they grew older. Nevertheless, in the early part of primary instruction it seems likely that the acquisition of numerical skills and writing ability could have been facilitated by the acceleration of finger recognition and other facets of psychomotor development (26).

A related concern is for an appropriate balance of physical and mental development. This can be traced back to the classical ideal of the "golden mean," the avoidance of excess in either physical or mental pursuits (151). The Greeks propounded the concept of "mens sana in corpore sano." In the words of Plato (79): "Music alone produces effeminacy, gymnastics alone produces ferocity, even savagery. Together, they produce harmony."

This insight was largely lost with the ascetic distortion of Christianity during the medieval period. Although some teachers of the Renaissance (da Feltre's l'umo universale) and the Enlightenment (Rousseau, Montaigne) recognized the unity of body and mind (122), physical activity is commonly regarded even today in instrumental terms—a reward, a diversion, or a means to improve athletic skills in order to enhance academic performance (151). Nevertheless, there is an increasing recognition of the interdependence of the body and the emotions (73), whether cognitive changes give rise to a physiological response (98) or vice versa (14). Even if affect and intelligence are seen as distinctive aspects of an individual's adaptation to his/her environment, they are complementary, inseparable, and undergo parallel development (29). Physical activity is critical to this development—in the words of Sherrington, "The muscle is the cradle of the recognizable mind" (*Man on his nature*, Cambridge Univer. Press, 1940). UNESCO has recognized this need in its official "Declaration on Sport" (International Council of Sport and Physical Education, UNESCO, 1964):

An individual, whatever his ultimate role in society, needs in his growing years a balance of intellectual, physical, moral and aesthetic development which must be reflected in the educational curriculum and timetable.

FOSTERING A HEALTHY LIFESTYLE

Few of the studies of physical activity in childhood have been followed up long enough to gauge their impact upon adult lifestyle. It would be encouraging to be able to demonstrate that a lifelong interest in physical activity had been generated, and that very few experimental students became addicted to cigarettes, alcohol, and drugs, but there is little unequivocal information on such issues.

Physical Activity

Although some educational theorists have maintained that an individual's attitudes are largely formed in early childhood, Leventhal (80) has argued that there is no strong evidence that children learn or act upon health information any more readily than adults. Indeed, if children are more readily molded, it might then be anticipated that a habit of daily activity formed early in life would persist into adulthood. Certainly, much depends upon the perceptions of physical activity formed during childhood.

Top-ranking young competitors are often required to train many hours per day to satisfy parents or coaches rather than any personal ambition. It is hardly surprising, then, that the ultimate impact upon physical activity is negative. Åstrand and his associates (8) found that within a few years of retiring from national competition Swedish female swimming champions had a lower level of maximum oxygen intake than the average Stockholm housewife of similar age. Likewise, Montoye et al. (90) noted that by middle-life, men who had earned an athletic letter at a university were taking less exercise and had gained more weight than others who had attended the same university without becoming involved in intercollegiate competition.

Required school programs may likewise have an adverse influence upon ultimate sports participation (94). Thus Rutenfranz and Lederle-Schenck (109) observed a virtual cessation of leisure activity in German adolescents when they moved from secondary school, where physical activity was required, to a vocational school, where it was not.

If the habit of regular physical activity is to persist into adult life, motivation must become internal. It cannot be dependent upon parent, coach, or schoolteacher. One criticism of competitive sport, with its external rewards, is that it tends to inhibit the development of such internal motivation (86). Moreover, it carries the seeds of its own demise. As a child becomes older, his/her interests apparently shift from competition to a recreational interpretation of physical activity (142); furthermore, as performance begins its inevitable age-related decline, the external rewards of competitive success and peer adulation progressively disappear. On the other hand, a cognitive internalization of the desired movement patterns does much to ensure lasting interest (130). A good instructor thus seeks not only to improve a child's performance but also to stress clearly the resulting implications for health.

Addictive Drugs

Most coaches actively discourage the use of socially abused and addictive drugs such as cigarettes, alcohol, and marijuana, and the students themselves are aware of the adverse effects of smoking or a hangover upon physical performance. Peer group pressure seems to be the most important factor influencing the behavior of the maturing child. The immediate effect of participating in vigorous physical activity is thus likely to be a decreased risk of initiating drug abuse. Unfortunately the advantage does not always persist when the sport is dropped. For example, Montoye et al. (90) found a higher proportion of cigarette smokers and heavy drinkers among former athletic letter holders than among other graduates of the same university. On the other hand, the proportion of smokers remains very low among adults who persist with endurance running (91) and cross-country skiing (63) into middle age. As with the habit of regular physical activity itself, the key to lifelong abstinence from drugs seems to be an internalization of motivation, with a clear understanding of the implications of behavior for future health. In this context, exercise becomes a useful positive component in a total health education package that inevitably contains quite a number of prohibitions.

IMPROVEMENT OF CURRENT HEALTH

Acute Disease

Little is known about the influence of physical activity upon the incidence of acute illness. The level of immune bodies in the blood is reputedly uninfluenced by physical activity. Athletic participation afforded an earlier generation no protection against tuberculosis, while it actually predisposed to the fulminant form of hepatitis and the paralytic form of anterior poliomyelitis (61).

Olympic contestants frequently request treatment for minor infections (61), yet this does not necessarily imply that vigorous exercise has increased susceptibility to disease. Other factors that increase the number of physician visits include exposure to unfamiliar microorganisms, swimming in polluted water (61), and anxiety about sustaining peak performance.

A recent controlled trial in Toronto suggested that introduction of an employee fitness program reduced the health costs of adult subjects by

$85 per person per year (123). Nevertheless, the savings apparently reflected an overall increase in health consciousness at the experimental company rather than a specific response to the augmented physical activity, since the benefit was demonstrated rather equally by participants and nonparticipants in the exercise classes.

Vitek et al. (148) examined the incidence of various diseases in 12- to 14-year-old boys, comparing control students both to recruits to specific sports programs and drop-outs from these programs. Considering all diseases, the attack rate was only insignificantly larger in control than in active students. When first recruited, ice hockey players had an above average incidence of diseases of the upper respiratory tract (acute tonsillitis, acute bronchitis, bronchiolitis, and influenza) but this disadvantage disappeared over 3 years of observation. Unfortunately, detailed statistics are not presented, although the authors concluded that the hockey-playing group developed "a rise in the resistance against the influences of cold medium."

The Trois-Rivières project (78) compared primary school attendance between children enrolled in a standard program of physical activity (one 40-minute period of physical activity per week) and those participating in an experimental program (5 hours of required physical activity per week). The first-grade experimental students were absent for 13 days, compared with 10 days for control students; in grades 2 through 6, both experimental and control students were absent for an average of 4 days per year. Possibly the younger students had not yet developed a full immunity to childhood diseases or were overprotected by anxious parents. If the latter supposition is correct, one could imagine an increase of protection when the parents realized that school attendance would involve an hour of physical activity. Certainly there was little evidence that increased activity influenced school attendance in either direction beyond grade 1.

Chronic Diseases

Physical activity is denied to many children because they suffer from some form of chronic disease. Many parents and physicians are overprotective, yet both immediate health and ultimate prognosis would be improved in many instances by participation in regular, graded physical activity programs (35,122).

The lesser degrees of congenital and acquired heart disease, including mild pulmonary stenosis, small atrial or ventricular septal defects, and mild mitral or aortic regurgitation are compatible with participation in all sports except those requiring very prolonged exercise (such as crosscountry running or skiing). More severe disorders (moderate pulmonary stenosis, moderate valve leaks, septal defects awaiting surgery, and most patients who have already undergone cardiac surgery) must be exercised with some caution, although many of these patients are also over-protected. A few of the most serious conditions such as incipient cardiac failure, cardiac dilation of more than 20%, acute myocardial disease, and a history of rheumatic fever during the past year are indications against participation in any type of physical education program (22,35,122).

Overprotection is common among children with asthmatic disorders (35). The fitness levels of such patients are suboptimal, and with a few exceptions (146) most reports indicate that they benefit greatly from vigorous training. Exercise seems particularly effective if it can be arranged in a residential setting away from the parents (117). Care must be taken to avoid inhaling cold, dry air since this can provoke an alarming exercise-induced bronchospasm (115). One of the most appropriate types of activity for the asthmatic child is swimming, and in some instances asthmatic individuals have advanced to the highest levels of international competition (37).

The most common childhood metabolic disorder among the developed nations is obesity. It remains debatable how much the moderate obesity characteristic of the North American teenager is a hazard to health (44). Observing obese children on film suggests that a low level of habitual activity is a major reason for the accumulation of body fat (87). This hypothesis is supported by physical working capacity values that are low with respect to body mass or heart volume (89). On the other hand, longitudinal observations suggest that increased physical education does little to correct established obesity while the student remains at home (126). The problem can be temporarily resolved in special residential camps, where vigorous activity is combined with rigorous dieting, but relapse is frequent once the child returns home (95).

Well controlled diabetes is compatible with normal participation in sports although care must be taken that the exercise bouts do not provoke an excessive rise in the concentrations of counter-regulatory and gluconeogenic hormones such as catecholamines, glucagon, growth hormone, and cortisol (68). A deliberate training program usually has a beneficial effect upon the course of the disease, sometimes to the point that insulin therapy is no longer required (68,69). Insulin sensitivity is enhanced, apparently because of increased binding of the hormone to receptors on the cell surface (69,97) rather than through an immediate usage of dietary glucose.

An increase of physical activity has a beneficial effect upon health in many chronic disorders of the central nervous system. With patience, considerable gains of physical ability can be induced in mentally retarded children (131). Improved working capacity is important to the functional health of such patients because most of them will ultimately need to support themselves in physically demanding occupations. As an added bonus (21,64) some, but not all (19), authors have reported gains of intellectual performance with training. Concerning cerebral palsy (96), a suitable conditioning program helps to correct a poor oxygen transporting power, a reduced cell mass, and increased body water (82). The benefit is derived in part from a stimulated appetite, although this is not the entire explanation since an equal response cannot be obtained by dietary supplements alone (13). For epilepsy, regular physical activity seems to raise the seizure threshold; the mechanism is unclear but one suggestion is that the effect is mediated through the release of lactic acid (22). The residual disability from a severe attack of anterior poliomyelitis is greatly reduced by an appropriate training program (137), although it remains unclear how much of the observed gains in performance reflect an enhanced self-image and a heightened sense of competition. Finally, the security and independence of children with sensory handicaps such as blindness can be developed through participation in activities that mimic the ideas and forms of normal sport (31).

Moderate degrees of kyphosis, scoliosis, and other posture defects (81,144) are of considerable concern to parents. Correction is often more for cosmetic than for functional reasons (103), although an improved appearance can enhance body image and resolve many minor aches and pains. Severe scoliosis leads to cardiorespiratory insufficiency and an associated limitation of physical working capacity (139), due primarily to a restrictive ventilatory defect (129). Recreation, endurance training (139), and specific muscle strengthening are all helpful forms of treatment, although the more severe spinal deformities often require surgery (139). Training allows an increase of alveolar ventilation, and the resulting improvement in ventilation/perfusion leads to increased oxygen transport.

PREVENTION OF FUTURE DISEASE

A number of the risk factors commonly associated with an increased incidence of cardiovascular disease in adults (an abnormal lipid profile, hypertension, cigarette smoking, physical inactivity, and obesity) are already present in a substantial proportion of North American school children (11). Deposition of fat in the lining of the larger arteries, for example, begins in infancy (15), and can be quite advanced in young adults (33). Serum cholesterol levels rise soon after birth, reaching adult levels within two years (12), although boys show a substantial decrease of total cholesterol at puberty (11). Blood pressures rise by about 1.7 mm Hg systolic and 0.7 mm Hg diastolic per year (12). Obesity affects some children from the early years of their schooling (118). Although 78% of U.S. students now recognize that cigarette smoking can cause lung cancer and is a factor in heart disease, the number of preadolescents who begin smoking shows little decline (59).

Risk factors tend to cluster in specific students. For example, abnormally high skinfold readings are associated with high blood pressure and high serum triglyceride readings. Moreover, in such individuals the adverse findings are relatively consistent from one year to the next (12,77). Thus it can be argued that the subjects concerned will continue to be at risk as adults; however, this is not necessarily true. Abraham et al. (2) followed 700 children from birth to adulthood and found that hypertension was associated with excess weight as adults but that the majority of those with high blood pressure had been below average weight as children!

The extent to which increased physical activity can normalize risk factors, and how far such normalization will improve a child's ultimate prognosis, also remains open to debate. The majority of young children with grossly abnormal lipid profiles probably have inherited disorders of fat metabolism (3,74). Likewise, some (133) but not all reports (51) have largely blamed childhood obesity upon inheritance rather than environmental factors such as diet and inactivity. Nevertheless, it remains likely that physical activity contributes to the prevention and control of several major risk factors. Thus Goldbloom (44) writes, "The one change in our children's lifestyle which might effect an ultimate reduction in the prevalence and severity of obesity and which would benefit the health of the entire population would be a significant increase in daily calorie expenditure. . . . Like other protective measures, it is most effective if initiated at the earliest possible age" (49).

AVOIDANCE OF INJURY

Health risks for the physically active child include acute effects upon the heart, the musculoskeletal system, and the psyche, plus more long-term influences upon health, attitudes, and personality.

Acute Cardiac Effects

Occasional distressing fatalities continue to occur in subjects performing vigorous sports (62). Rose (107) noted that 24 of 44 sudden deaths in athletes occurred in subjects under 17 years of age. Spurious calculations once purported to show that the great blood vessels failed to grow in proportion to other parts of the body, placing the heart and circulation of the young child under a dangerous strain during hard physical exertion (52). We now know that such fears are groundless. Fatigue causes a healthy child to stop exercising long before any danger point is reached (70) and, furthermore, the child is at no particular anatomical disadvantage relative to the adult. A fair proportion of emergencies arise from congenital anomalies such as aortic stenosis, aberrant coronary vessels, and berry aneurysms of the Circle of Willis. Better pediatric examination would diagnose some of these problems, but in the absence of invasive testing such as coronary arteriography (108) other problems will inevitably remain silent until a catastrophe occurs. Since such children are in any event likely to succumb to their abnormality at a relatively early age, the hazard of "silent" cardiovascular disease can hardly be an argument for a general prohibition of physical activity in childhood. Indeed, it is probably preferable that any critical incidents should develop when the individual is exercising under supervision rather than when playing on his or her own.

Acute viral infections are an important contraindication to both vigorous training and competition. There is a danger of myocarditis, leading to cardiac damage and a fatal heart block or fibrillation (71). Unfortunately the cardiac infection is not always detected by routine electrocardiography, and the only safe course is to forbid strenuous exercise whenever a child has a viral illness.

Musculoskeletal Disorders

The child who engages in vigorous sport or recreation faces a much greater risk of mechanical injury than of cardiovascular problems. The incidence of musculoskeletal disorders remains far too high in most childhood sports (41). Data from four high schools in the Seattle area (41) showed U.S. football and wrestling to be the two most dangerous pursuits, with 506 of 624 participants sustaining football injuries and 176 of 234 sustaining wrestling injuries over a one-year season.

A health maintenance organization in the New York area found that 1.7% of all pediatric visits were attributable to sports injuries, football and skateboarding being the prime culprits; nevertheless, the practical difficulty of prevention is evident in that more than 50% of accidents occurred during unsupervised play (43). Finally, reports for Czechoslovakia show that physical education and sports together accounted for 8 to 11% of all recorded accidents (58), with 0.5% of 10- to 14-year-old students suffering injury during the required physical education classes (54).

One very common condition among child athletes is traumatic epiphysitis. Adams (5) found lesions of the medial epicondyle in all 80 of a group of Little League baseball pitchers, whereas only a few nonpitching players showed any abnormalities. Similar problems can develop in the tibial tubercle of the young runner or jumper (75). The best clinical approach is to avoid the condition through (a) less severe competition and (b) careful examination of any competitor who reports pain in a vulnerable area.

Because ossification of a child's long bones is still incomplete, minor twists and tumbles can cause fractures that would not occur in an adult.

More seriously, 10 to 15% of fractures involve the growing epiphyseal plate, and in 10 to 20% of such epiphyseal injuries growth of the bone is subsequently distorted (1,75). Factors contributing to the likelihood of injury include too heavy a training volume and an excessive level of competition (104). Players should be matched for size and skill, as well as for age, and should be encouraged to compete against themselves rather than against stronger rivals.

Psychological Effects

The psychological pressures of intense competition are particularly undesirable in a young performer (102,147). Some reports have described a substantial excretion of catecholamines during contests (16), with participants too excited to eat or sleep (42,132). Nevertheless, there is a relatively rapid recovery to a normal resting heart rate (50-132). Rivard et al. (106) examined students who were participating in a provincial ice hockey championship. Classroom teachers placed 88% of participants in the upper half of the class before competition, and 82% remained in this category when they returned to school. Scores for motivation, group integration, school attendance, and obedience were all favorable relative to other pupils, while scores on a test of frustration remained unaltered, regardless of whether the team won or lost. It would thus appear that although competition causes some immediate excitement for the child, the effects of a regional or a provincial competition are relatively short lived.

Long-Term Health Effects

Possible effects upon cardiovascular health have already been considered. An exercise program that is continued into adult life is likely to have a beneficial influence upon long-term health. However, the star sports performers too often cease all activity once their performance begins to decline. Their health status may then be worse than that of a sedentary individual (92), particularly if the heart volume was increased by the original training program (53 but not 101 or 110).

Sports' long-term impact upon attitudes and behavior merits further examination. Some authors have described a catharsis of emotions and a release of tension and stress, but others believe that excessive competition and a culture of violence have an adverse influence upon the child's overall psychological development (119).

CONCLUSIONS

There remains a need for physicians and physical educators to devote more attention to the wellness of the growing child. An increase of physical activity apparently has relatively little influence upon physical development but it can speed psychomotor development and thus boost academic progress. The long-term impact depends very much upon the type of program adopted. A favorable lifestyle may be inculcated at an early age but undue compulsion can detract from motivation. Physical activity has little influence upon the risk of acute illness; however, it is beneficial in chronic cardiovascular disease, respiratory disease, certain metabolic disorders, and neurological disorders. By controlling the evolution of certain risk factors, exercise may also protect against future disease. In order to maximize benefits, it is important to guard against certain acute and long-term hazards of vigorous activity including sudden cardiac death, various potential musculoskeletal disorders, and psychological hazards. A program of enhanced activity not only favors wellness, but also seems important to the well balanced development of the child.

REFERENCES

1. Abraham, E., A. Ansari, and T.L. Huang. Fracture of distal medial femoral epiphysis with subluxation of the knee joint. *J. Trauma*, 20:339-341, 1980.

2. Abraham, S., G. Collins, and M. Nordsiech. Relationship of childhood weight status to morbidity in adults. *Publ. Hlth. Rep.*, 86:273-284, 1971.

3. Abrahams, P.H., H.G. Schrott, W.R. Clarke, and R.M. Lauer. "Prevalence of fatal coronary artery disease in relatives of hypertriglyceridemic school children." In *Atherosclerosis* IV, edited by G. Schettler, Y. Goto, Y. Hata, and G. Klose, p. 506. Berlin: Springer Verlag, 1977.

4. Adams, E.H. A comparative anthropometric study of hard labor during youth as a stimulator of physical growth of young colored women. *Res. Quart.*, 9:102, 1938.

5. Adams, J.E. Bone injuries in very young athletes. *Clin. Orthop.*, 58:129-140, 1968.

6. American Public Health Assoc. *Health supervision of young children*. New York: American Public Health Association, 1954.

7. Andrew, G.M., M.R. Becklake, J.S. Guleria, and D.V. Bates. Heart and lung functions in swimmers and non-athletes during growth. *J. Appl. Physiol.*, 32:245-251, 1972.

8. Åstrand, P.O., L. Engström, B. Eriksson, P. Karlberg, I. Nylander, B. Saltin, and C. Thorén. Girl swimmers. With special reference to respiratory and circulatory adaptation and gynaecological and psychiatric aspects. *Acta Paediatr.*, 147 (Suppl.):1-75, 1963.

9. Bailey, D.A. "Exercise, fitness and physical education for the growing child." In *Proceedings of the National Conference on Fitness and*

Health, edited by W.A.R. Orban, pp. 13-27. Ottawa: Health & Welfare Canada, 1973.

10. Bar Or, O. and L.D. Zwiren. "Physiological effects of increased frequency of physical education classes and of endurance conditioning on 9 to 10-year-old girls and boys." In *Pediatric work physiology.* Proceedings of 4th International Symposium, edited by O. Bar Or, pp. 183-198. Natanya, Israel: Wingate Institute, 1973.

11. Berenson, G.S., S.R. Srinivasan, A.W. Voors, and L.S. Webber. "Clues to mechanisms of cardiovascular disease from an epidemiologic study of children—The Bogalusa Heart Study." In *Atherosclerosis* V, edited by A.M. Gotto, L.C. Smith, and B. Allen, pp. 272-277. Berlin: Springer Verlag, 1980.

12. Berenson, G.S., L.S. Webber, S.R. Srinivasan, R.R. Frerichs, and A.W. Voors. "Inter-relationships and persistence of risk factor variables at high levels in children—The Bogalusa Heart Study." In *International Conference on Atherosclerosis*, edited by L.A. Carlson, R. Paolett, C.R. Sirtori, and G. Weber, pp. 357-364. New York: Raven Press, 1978.

13. Berg, K. Remarks on physical training of children with cerebral palsy. *Acta Physiol. Scand.,* 217 (Suppl.):106-107, 1971.

14. Bindra, D. A unified interpretation of emotion and motivation. *Ann. N.Y. Acad. Sci.,* 159:1071-1083, 1961.

15. Blieden, L.C., and N. Neufeld. "Morphologic aspects of childhood atherosclerosis." In *Atherosclerosis* IV, edited by G. Schettler, Y. Goto, Y. Hata, and G. Klose, pp. 498-505. Berlin: Springer Verlag, 1977.

16. Blimkie, C.J., D.A. Cunningham, and Y.F. Leung. "Urinary catecholamine excretion and lactate concentrations in competitive hockey players aged 11 to 23 years." In *Frontiers of activity and child health*, edited by H. Lavallée and R.J. Shephard, pp. 313-321. Quebec City: Editions du Pélican, 1977.

17. Brown, C.H., J.R. Harrower, and M.F. Deeter. The effects of cross-country running on pre-adolescent girls. *Med. Sci. Sports*, 4:1-5, 1972.

18. Campbell, W.R., and R.H. Pohndorf. "Physical fitness of British and United States children." In *Report of conference on health and fitness in the modern world*, edited by L.A. Larson, pp. 8-16. Chicago: Athletic Institute, 1961.

19. Chasey, W.C., and W. Wyrick. Effect of a gross motor developmental program on form perception skills of educable mentally retarded children. *Res. Quart.,* 41:345-352, 1970.

20. Clarke, H.H. Athletes. Their academic achievement and personal-social status. President's Council on Physical Fitness and Sport. *Phys. Fitness Res. Digest,* 5(3):1-23, 1975.

21. Cratty, B.J. *Motor activity and education of retardates*. Philadelphia: Lea & Febiger, 1969.

22. Cumming, G.R. Le sport chez les enfants affectés de troubles cardiaques, d'asthme ou d'epilepsie. *Vie Méd. Can. Fr.,* 4:347-354, 1975.

23. Cumming, G.R., A Goodwin, G. Baggley, and J. Antel. Repeated measurements of aerobic capacity during a week of intensive training at a youth's track camp. *Canad. J. Physiol. Pharmacol.,* 45:805-811, 1967.

24. Cumming, G.R., D. Goulding, and G. Baggley. Failure of school physical education to improve cardiorespiratory fitness. *Canad. Med. Assoc. J.,* 101:69-73, 1969.

25. Cumming, G.R., and R. Keynes. A fitness performance test for school children and its correlation with physical working capacity and maximal oxygen uptake. *Canad. Med. Assoc. J.,* 96:1262-1269, 1967.

26. Curcio, F., O. Robbins, and S. Ela. The role of body parts and readiness in acquisition of number conservation. *Child Dev.,* 42:1641-1646, 1971.

27. Dalton, K. Menstruation and examinations. *Lancet,* 2:1386-1388, 1968.

28. Daum, W. "The main features of present-day society." In *Child in sport and physical activity*, edited by J.G. Albinson and G. Andrew, pp. 3-18. Baltimore: University Park Press, 1976.

29. Decarie, T. "Affect development and cognition in a Piagetian context." In *The development of affect*, edited by M. Lewis and L. Rosenblum, pp. 183-204. New York: Plenum, 1978.

30. Dietrich, R., C. Kiess, P. Schenderlein, et al. Die Trainierbarkeit von Jugendlichen im Alter von 14 bis 19 Jahren. *Med. Sport,* 14:142-147, 1974.

31. Dordel, H.J. "Physical education and sport for the visually handicapped and blind." In *Sport as a means of rehabilitation*, edited by U. Simri, pp. 9/1-9/10. Natanya, Israel: Wingate Institute, 1970.

32. Ekblöm, B. Effect of physical training on adolescent boys. *J. Appl. Physiol.,* 27:350-355, 1969.

33. Enos, W.F., J.C. Bayer, and R.H. Holmes. Pathogenesis of coronary disease in American soldiers killed in Korea. *J. Amer. Med. Assoc.,* 158:912-914, 1955.

34. Eriksson, B.O. Physical training, oxygen supply and muscle metabolism in 11- 13-year-old boys. *Acta Physiol. Scand.,* 384 (Suppl.):1-48, 1972.

35. Eriksson, B.O. "The child in sport and physical activity—medical aspects." In *Child in sport and physical activity*, edited by J.G. Albinson and G.M. Andrew, pp. 43-65. Baltimore: University Park Press, 1976.

36. Fabricius, H. Effect of added calisthenics on the physical fitness of fourth grade boys and girls. *Res. Quart.,* 35:135-140, 1964.

37. Fitch, K.D. "Swimming medicine and asthma." In *Swimming*

medicine IV, edited by B. Eriksson and B. Furberg, pp. 16-31. Baltimore: University Park Press, 1978.

38. Franks, D.B., and G.C. Moore. Effects of calisthenics and volleyball on the AAHPER fitness test and volleyball skill. *Res. Quart.*, 40:288-292, 1969.

39. Frisch, R.E., and J.W. McArthur. Menstrual cycles. Fatness as a determinant of minimum for their maintenance or onset. *Science*, 185:949-951, 1974.

40. Frisch, R.E., G. Wyshak, and L. Vincent. Delayed menarche and amenorrhoea in ballet dancers. *New Engl. J. Med.*, 303:17-19, 1980.

41. Garrick, J.G., and R.K. Requa. Injuries in high school sports. *Pediatrics*, 61:465-469, 1978.

42. Giddings, G.A. "Sleep in children. A report of the joint committee on health problems in education of NEA and AMA, 1956." Cited by G.L. Rarick. In *Physical activity: Human growth and development*, edited by G.L. Rarick, p. 386. New York: Academic Press, 1973.

43. Goldberg, G., P.A. Witman, G.W. Gleim, and J.A. Nicholas. Children's sports injuries: Are they avoidable? *Phys. Sports Med.*, 7:93-101, 1979.

44. Goldbloom, R.B. "Obesity in childhood." In *The child and physical activity*, edited by R.C. Goode and R. Volpe, pp. 55-70. Toronto: Ont. Heart Foundation, 1979.

45. Goode, R.C., A. Virgin, T.T. Romet, D. Crawford, J. Duffin, T. Pollandi, and Z. Woch. Effects of a short period of physical activity in adolescent boys and girls. *Can. J. Appl. Sports Sci.*, 1:241-250, 1976.

46. Gordon, E.E., K. Kowalski, and M. Fritts. Changes in rat muscle fiber with forceful exercises. *Arch. Phys. Med. Rehabil.*, 48: 577-582, 1967.

47. Gruber, J.J. Exercise and mental performance. *Int. J. Sport Psychol.*, 6:28-40, 1975.

48. Hammett, V.B.O. "Physiological changes with physical training." In International Symposium on Physical Activity and Cardiovascular Health. *Canad. Med. Assoc. J.*, 96:764-768, 1967.

49. Hanefeld, M., W. Leonhardt, and H. Haller. "Coronary risk factors in adults: The influence of nutrition in early life." In *Atherosclerosis* IV, edited by G. Schettler, Y. Goto, Y. Hata, and G. Klose, pp. 104-108. Berlin: Springer Verlag, 1977.

50. Hanson, D.L. Cardiac response to participation in Little League baseball competition as determined by telemetry. *Res. Quart.*, 38:384-388, 1967.

51. Hewitt, D. Sib resemblance in bone, muscle and fat measurements of the human calf. *Ann. Hum. Genet.*, 22:213-221, 1958.

52. Hollman, W. Der Arbeits und Trainingseinfluss auf Kreislauf und Atmung. Darmstadt: Steinkopff Verlag, 1959.

53. Holmgren, A., and T. Strandell. Relationship between heart

volume, total haemoglobin and physical work capacity in former athletes. *Acta Med. Scand.*, 163:146-160, 1959.

54. Hornof, Z. "Obecné zásady prevence úrazú v tělesné výchově." In *Télovychovne lékǎrstvi*, edited by J. Král, pp. 249-255. SZDN: Praha, 1969.

55. Hunsicker, P.A. *American Assoc. for Health, Physical Education and Recreation youth fitness test manual. Testing methods and norms.* Washington, DC: AAHPER, 1958.

56. Hunsicker, P., and G. Reiff. AAHPER youth fitness test manual. (Revised edition.) Washington, DC: AAHPER, 1976.

57. Ilmarinen, J., and J. Rutenfranz. "Longitudinal studies of the changes in habitual physical activity of schoolchildren and working adolescents." In *Children and exercise* IX, edited by K. Berg and B. Eriksson, pp. 149-159. Baltimore: University Park Press, 1980.

58. Jánošdeák, J., L. Komandel, and M. Palat. Traumatologiá a prvá pomoc pre poslucháčov telesnej výchovy. Slovenské pedagog. naklad., Bratislava, Slovakia, 1965.

59. Jesse, M.J. "Cigarette smoking: A risk factor for atherosclerosis in childhood?" In *Atherosclerosis* V, edited by A.M. Gotto, L.C. Smith, and B. Allen, pp. 278-281. Berlin: Springer Verlag, 1980.

60. Johnson, E.L. Effects of 5-day-a-week versus 2- and 3-day-a-week physical education class on fitness skill, adipose tissue and growth. *Res. Quart.*, 40:93-98, 1969.

61. Jokl, E. "The immunological status of athletes." In *The role of exercise in internal medicine*, edited by D. Brunner and E. Jokl, pp. 129-134. Basel: Karger, 1977.

62. Jokl, E., and J.T. McClellan. Exercise and cardiac death. Baltimore: University Park Press, 1971.

63. Karvonen, M.J., H. Klemola, J. Virkajärvi, and A. Kekkonen. Longevity of endurance skiers. *Med. Sci. Sports*, 6:49-51, 1974.

64. Kasch, F.W., and S.A. Zasueta. Physical capacities of mentally retarded children. *Acta Paediatr. Scand.*, 217 (Suppl.):114-118, 1971.

65. Kato, S., and T. Ishiko. "Obstructed growth of children's bones due to excessive labor in remote corners." In *Proceedings of International Congress of Sports Sciences*, 1964, edited by K. Kato, p. 479. Tokyo: Japanese Union of Sports Sciences, 1966.

66. Kemper, H.C.G., R. Verschuur, K.J.A. Ras, J. Suel, P.G. Splinter, L.W.C. Tavecchio, and R. Verschuur. "Investigation into the effects of two extra physical education lessons per week during one school year upon the physical development of 12- and 13-year-old boys." In *Pediatric work physiology*, edited by J. Borms and M. Hebbelinck, pp. 159-166. Basel: Karger, 1978.

67. Knuttgen, H.G. Comparison of fitness of Danish and American schoolchildren. *Res. Quart.*, 32:190-196, 1961.

68. Koivistio, V.A., and L. Groop. "Prognostic significance of physi-

cal training in juvenile diabetes." In *Physical training in health promotion and medial care*, edited by O. Hänninen, K. Kukkonen, and I. Vuori. *Ann. Clin. Res.*, 14 (Suppl. 34):74-79, 1982.

69. Koivisto, V.A., and R.S. Sherwin. Exercise in Diabetes — therapeutic implications. *Post Grad. Med.*, 66:87-96, 1979.

70. Komadel, L. "Vplyv sportovej pripravy na zdravie, morfologický a funkčný vývoj mládeže." In *Acta Fac. Educ. Phys. Univ. Comenianae.*, 10:193-214, 1971.

71. Koplan, P. Cardiovascular deaths while running. *J. Amer. Med. Assoc.*, 242:2578-2579, 1979.

72. Kraus, H., and R.P. Hirschland. Minimum muscular fitness tests in schoolchildren. *Res. Quart.*, 25:178-187, 1954.

73. Krech, D. "Does behaviour really need a brain?" In *William James: Unfinished business*, edited by R.B. MacLeod, pp. 1-11. Washington, DC: American Psychological Association, 1969.

74. Kwiterovich, P.O. "Pediatric lipoprotein metabolism and atherosclerosis: A prospectus." In *Atherosclerosis V*, edited by A.M. Gotto, L.C. Smith, and B. Allen, pp. 286-293. Berlin: Springer Verlag, 1980.

75. Larson, R.L. "Physical activity and the growth and development of bone and joint structures." In *Physical activity, human growth and development*, edited by G.L. Rarick, pp. 33-59. New York: Academic Press, 1973.

76. Laska-Mierzejewska, T. "Body build as one of the elements of selection and adaptation of competitors in team games." In *Kinanthropometry* II, edited by M. Ostyn, G. Beunen, J. Simons, pp. 214-221. Baltimore: University Park Press, 1980.

77. Lauer, R.M., and W.R. Clarke. "Tracking of coronary risk factors in children: The Muscatine study." In *Atherosclerosis V*, edited by A.M. Gotto, L.C. Smith, and B. Allen, pp. 294-301. Berlin: Springer Verlag, 1980.

78. Lavallée, H., and R.J. Shephard. *Croissance et développement*. Trois Rivières: Université de Québec, 1982.

79. Lee, H. (Translator). *Plato: Timaeus and Cortias*. London, England: Penguin Books, 1971.

80. Leventhal, H. Changing attitudes and habits to reduce risk factors in chronic diseases. *Amer. J. Cardiol.*, 31:571-580, 1973.

81. Lonstein, J.E., R.B. Winter, J.H. Moe, et al. School screening for the early detection of spine deformities. Progress and pitfalls. *Minn. Med.*, 59:51-57, 1976.

82. Lundberg, A., and B. Pernow. The effect of physical training on blood flow through exercising muscle in adolescents with motor handicaps. *Scand. J. Clin. Lab. Invest.*, 26:89-96, 1970.

83. Maigre, A., and J. Destroper. *L'education psychomotrice*. Paris: Presses Universitaires de France, 1975.

84. Martens, F.L. *The Cordova Bay Project*. Unpublished report to

University of Victoria (see Volpe, ref. 151).

85. Martens, F.L. Personality, attitudes and academic achievement of athletic and non-athletic junior high school boys. *Percept. Mot. Skills*, 39:538, 1974.

86. Martens, R. "Competitiveness in sports." In *Physical activity and human well-being*, edited by F. Landry and W.A.R. Orban, pp. 323-344. Miami, FL: Symposia Specialists, 1978.

87. Mayer, J. Inactivity as a major factor in adolescent obesity. *Ann. N.Y. Acad. Sci.*, 131:502-506, 1965.

88. McCammon, R.W. *Human growth and development*. Springfield, IL: C.C. Thomas, 1970.

89. Mocellin, R., and J. Rutenfranz. Investigations of the physical working capacity of obese children. *Acta Paediatr. Scand.*, 217:77-79, 1971.

90. Montoye, H.J., W.D. Van Huss, H.W. Olson, W.O. Pierson, and A.J. Hudec. *The longevity and morbidity of college athletes*. Michigan State University, East Lansing: Phi Epsilon Kappa Fraternity, 1957.

91. Morgan, P., M. Gildiner, and G.R. Wright. Smoking reduction in adults who take up exercise: A survey of a running club for adults. *CAHPER Journal*, 42:39-43, 1976.

92. Murayama, M., and V. Kuroda. "Cardiovascular future of athletes." In *Sports cardiology*, edited by T. Lubich and A. Venerando, pp. 401-414. Bologna: Aulo Gaggi, 1980.

93. Noguchi, Y. *A comparative study of motor fitness between Japanese and American youth*. Tokyo: Ministry of Education, 1960.

94. Novák, A., H. Střelcová, H. Němcová, and F. Salajka. "Biosocial environment and psychologic development." In *Youth and Physical Activity*, edited by Z. Placheta, pp. 37-54. Brno: J.E. Purkyne University, 1980.

95. Pařízková, J. *Body fat and physical fitness*. The Hague: M. Nijhoff, 1977.

96. Pearson, P.H., and C.E. Williams. *Physical therapy services in the developmental disabilities*. Springfield, IL: C.C. Thomas, 1972.

97. Pedersen, O., H. Beck-Nielsen, and L. Heding. Increased insulin receptors after exercise in patients with insulin-dependent Diabetes Mellitus. *New Engl. J. Med.*, 302:886-892, 1980.

98. Persky, H. Adrenocortical function and anxiety. *Psychoneuroendocrinology*, 1:37-44, 1975.

99. Phillips, M.A., C. Bookwalter, C. Denman, J. McAuley, H. Sherwin, D. Summers, and H. Yeakel. Analysis of results from the Kraus-Weber tests of minimum muscular fitness in children. *Res. Quart.*, 26:314-323, 1955.

100. Piaget, J. Motricité, perception et intelligence. *Enfance*, 9:9-14, 1956.

101. Pyorala, K., M.J. Karvonen, P. Taskinen, J. Takkunen and H.

Kyronseppa. "Cardiovascular studies on former endurance athletes." In *Physical activity and the heart*, edited by M.J. Karvonen and A.J. Barry, pp. 301-310. Springfield, IL: C.C. Thomas, 1967.

102. Rarick, G.L., ed. "Competitive sports in childhood and early adolescence." In *Physical activity: Human growth and development*. New York: Academic Press, 1973.

103. Rathbone, J.L. "Good posture, the expression of good development." In *Symposium on posture, Phi Delta Pi*, 1938 (Cited by D.K. Matthews, Measurement in physical education. Philadelphia: Lea & Febiger, 1963.)

104. Reeves, J.S.H., and S.W. Mendryk. "A study of the incidence, nature and cause of hockey injuries in the greater Edmonton metropolitan area." In *Application of science and medicine to sport*, edited by A.W. Taylor, pp. 301-308. Springfield, IL: C.C. Thomas, 1975.

105. Ring, G.C. , M. Bosch, and L. Chu-Shek. Effects of exercise on growth, resting metabolism and body composition of Fischer rats. *Biol. Med.*, 133:1162-1165, 1970.

106. Rivard, G., H. Lavallée, M. Rajic et al. "Influence of competitive hockey on physical condition and psychological behaviour of children." In *Frontiers of activity and child health*, edited by H. Lavallée and R.J. Shephard, pp. 335-354. Quebec City: Editions du Pélican, 1977.

107. Rose, K.D. Relationship of cardiac problems to athletic participation. *J. Amer. Med. Assoc.*, 208:2319-2324, 1969.

108. Rose, K.D. The potential for cardiovascular accidents in athletes with a heart problem. *Med. Sci. Sports*, 1:144-151, 1969.

109. Rutenfranz, J., and U. Lederle-Schenk. School sport and sporting interests upon growing up (in German). *Die Berliner Arztekammer*, 5:408-410, 1968. (Cited by Ilmarinen and Rutenfranz, ref. 57)

110. Saltin, B., and G. Grimby. Physiological analysis of middle-aged and old former athletes. Comparison of still active athletes of the same ages. *Circulation*, 38:1104-1115, 1968.

111. Schneider, E. *Physical education in urban elementary schools*. Washington, DC: U.S. Office of Education, 1961.

112. Schuck, G.R. Effects of athletic competition on growth and development of junior high school boys. *Res. Quart.*, 33:288-298, 1962.

113. Selye, H. *The stress of life*. New York: McGraw-Hill, 1956.

114. Shephard, R.J. *Endurance fitness* (2nd edition). Toronto: University of Toronto Press, 1977.

115. Shephard, R.J. Exercise-induced bronchospasm. A review. *Med. Sci. Sports*, 9: 1-10, 1977.

116. Shephard, R.J. *Human physiological work capacity*. London: Cambridge University Press, 1978.

117. Shephard, R.J. Exercise for the asthmatic patient—a brief historical review. *J. Sports Med. Phys. Fitness*, 18:301-307, 1978.

118. Shephard, R.J. "Fitness, obesity and health." In *Proceedings of First RSG4 Physical Fitness Symposium with special reference to military forces*, edited by C. Allen, pp. 238-261. Downsview, Ont: Defence & Civil Inst. Env. Med., 1978.

119. Shephard, R.J. *The fit athlete*. London: Oxford University Press, 1978.

120. Shephard, R.J. Ischaemic heart disease and physical activity. London: Croom-Helm, 1981.

121. Shephard, R.J., Presidential address. In *Croissance et développement*, edited by H. Lavallée and R.J. Shephard, pp. 29-43. Trois Rivières: Université de Québec, 1982.

122. Shephard, R.J. Physical activity and growth. Chicago: Year Book Publications, 1982.

123. Shephard, R.J., P. Corey, P. Renzland, and M. Cox. The influence of an employee fitness and lifestyle modification programme upon medical care costs. *Canad. J. Publ. Health*, 73:259-263, 1982.

124. Shephard, R.J., H. Lavallée, J.C. Jéquier, M. Rajic, and C. Beaucage. "Un programme complémentaire d'éducation physique. Etude préliminaire de l'expérience pratiquée dans le district de Trois Rivières." In *Facteurs limitant l'endurance humaine. Les techniques d'amélioration de la performance*, edited by J.R. LaCour, pp. 43-54. Université de St. Etienne, France, 1977.

125. Shephard, R.J., H. Lavallée, J.C. Jéquier, R. LaBarre, M. Rajic, and C. Beaucage. "Seasonal differences in aerobic power." In *Physical fitness assessment — Principles, practice and application*, edited by R.J. Shephard and H. Lavallée, pp. 194-210. Springfield, IL: C.C. Thomas, 1978.

126. Shephard, R.J., H. Lavallée, J.C. Jéquier, R. LaBarre, and M. Rajic. A community approach to assessments of exercise tolerance in health and disease. *J. Sports Med. Phys. Fitness*, 19:297-304, 1979.

127. Shephard, R.J., H. Lavallée, and G. Larivière. Competitive selection among age-class ice-hockey players. *Brit. J. Sports Med.*, 12:11-13, 1978.

128. Shephard, R.J., H. Lavallée, M. Rajic, J.C. Jéquier, G. Brisson, and C. Beaucage. "Radiographic age in the interpretation of physiological and anthropological data." In *Pediatric work physiology*, edited by J. Borms and M. Hebbelinck, pp. 124-133. Basel: Karger, 1978.

129. Shneerson, J.M. Cardiac and respiratory responses to exercise in adolescent idiopathic scoliosis. *Thorax*, 35:347-350, 1980.

130. Silvennoinen, M. On the principles of developing and comparing objective and content structures in physical education with special reference to the Finnish comprehensive school curriculum. Jyväskalä. *Rep. Phys. Culture Health*, 24:9-18, 1979.

131. Skrobak-Kaczynski, J., and T. Varik. "Physical fitness and trainability of young male patients with Down Syndrome." In *Children*

and exercise IX, edited by K. Berg and B. O. Eriksson, pp. 300-316. Baltimore: University Park Press, 1980.

132. Skubic, E. Emotional responses of boys to little-league and middle-league competitive baseball. *Res. Quart.*, 26:342-352, 1955.

133. Slack, J., M. Preece, and P. Giles. "Identification of children who are heterozygotes for familial hypercholesterolaemia." In *Atherosclerosis* V, edited by A.M. Gotto, L.C. Smith, and B. Allen, pp. 244-247. Berlin: Springer Verlag, 1980.

134. Sloan, A.W. Physical fitness of South African compared with British and American high school children. *S. Afr. Med. J.*, 40:688-690, 1966.

135. Sorochan, W.D. Health concepts as a basis for orthobiosis. *J. School Health*, 38:673-682, 1968.

136. Spence, J., W.S. Walton, F.J.W. Miller, and S.D.M. Court. *A thousand families in Newcastle Upon Tyne. An approach to the study of health and illness in children.* London: Oxford University Press, 1954.

137. Spira, R. "Physical impact of sport activities in a group of post-poliomyelitic paralytic subjects." In *Sport as a means of rehabilitation*, edited by U. Simri, pp. 3/1-3/14. Natanya, Israel: Wingate Institute, 1970.

138. Stewart, K.J., and B. Gutin. Effects of physical training on cardiorespiratory fitness in children. *Res. Quart.*, 47:110-120, 1976.

139. Stoboy, H. "Pulmonary function and spiroergometric criteria in scoliotic patients before and after Harrington rod surgery and physical exercise." In *Pediatric work physiology*, edited by J. Borms and M. Hebbelinck, pp. 72-81. Baltimore: University Park Press. 1978.

140. Strydom, N.B. "Environmental variables affecting fitness testing." In *Physical fitness assessment. Principles, practice and application*, edited by H. Lavallée and R.J. Shephard, pp. 94-101. Springfield, IL: C.C. Thomas, 1978.

141. Tanner, J.M. *The physique of the Olympic athlete.* London: Unwin, 1964.

142. Telama, R., and M. Silvennoinen. Structure and development of 11- to 19-year-olds: Motivation for physical activity. *Scand. J. Sports Sci.*, 1:23-31, 1979.

143. Terrisse, B., and L. Allard. Education psychomotrice, développement et apprentissage scolaire. *Mouvement*, 10:25-30, 1975.

144. Turner, M. *Faulty posture and its treatment.* London: Whitefriars Press, 1965.

145. Varstala, V., R. Telama, and O. Akkanen. "Teacher and pupil activities during physical education lessons." In *Proc. 12th Int. Congress of ICHPER*, pp. 1-7. Cited in *Research in Physical Culture in Finland*. Finnish Society for Research in Sports and Physical Education. Publication 16:35, 1979.

146. Vávra, J., M. Mácek, B. Mrzena, and V. Spicák. Intensive physi-

cal training in children with bronchial asthma. *Acta Paediatr. Scand.,* 217 (Suppl.):90-92, 1971.

147. Vaz, E.W. "The culture of young hockey players." In *Training — Scientific basis and application,* edited by A.W. Taylor, pp. 222-234. Springfield, IL: C.C. Thomas, 1972.

148. Vitek, D., D. Blahová, and K. Dominková. "State of health." In *Youth and physical activity,* edited by Z. Placheta, pp. 55-60. Brno: J.E. Purkyné Universitat, 1980.

149. Volle, M., R.J. Shephard, H. Lavallée, R. LaBarre, J.C. Jéquier, and M. Rajic. "Influence of a programme of required physical activity upon academic performance." In *Croissance et développement,* edited by H. Lavallée and R.J. Shephard, pp. 91-108. Trois Rivières: Université de Québec, 1982.

150. Volle, M., H. Tisal, R. LaBarre, H. Lavallée, R.J. Shephard, J.C. Jéquier, and M. Rajic. "Influence d'un programme expérimental d'activités physiques integré a l'école primaire sur le développement de quelques élements psychomoteurs." In *Croissance et développement,* edited by H. Lavallée and R.J. Shephard, pp. 201-219. Trois Rivières: Université de Québec, 1982.

151. Volpe, R. "Physical activity, intellectual and emotional development." In *The child and physical activity,* edited by R.C. Goode and R. Volpe, pp. 84-102. Toronto: Ontario Heart Foundation, 1979.

152. Wireman, E.O. Comparison of four approaches to increasing physical fitness. *Res. Quart.,* 31:658-666, 1960.

153. World Health Organization. *Constitution of the World Health Organization.* Chronicle of WHO, 1:1-2, 1947.

2

Body Composition
in Children and Youth[1]

Timothy G. Lohman, Richard A. Boileau,
and Mary H. Slaughter
University of Illinois

Quantification and evaluation of body composition are essential when considering the growth and maturation of children. Further, the assessment of nutritional status, including obesity and underweight conditions, can be more accurately assessed by defining the composition of body weight. Body weight can be partitioned into its basic compositional components of fat and fat-free body weight or lean body mass. While body weight is often used alone or in combination with age, height, and frame size to estimate ideal weight, such methods do not address the relative composition or quality of the body weight. With improved detection and awareness of the problems related to childhood obesity as well as other

[1]The research and literature review was supported in part by NIH Grant Am 26351.

nutrition and metabolic related diseases of children, it is important that practitioners understand the conceptual basis of body composition assessment so that they can appropriately interpret fatness and leanness. This chapter reviews the conventional methods of measuring body composition in children, including the limitations and assumptions of present methods in relation to the apparent chemical immaturity of children.

Research on body composition in children and youth, and the influence of exercise and various environmental factors on changes in body composition in growing children, are based on indirect methods rather than the direct measurement of lean and fat tissue. Critical to most indirect methods is the assumption that the fat-free (FFB) body does not change significantly in its composition during growth and development. Considerable evidence based on several animal species indicates that after puberty the fat-free body composition stabilizes and remains relatively constant for a considerable period of adult life before changes associated with senescence occur. For humans, stabilization of the fat-free body composition has not been verified.

Moulton (54) first formulated the concept of chemical maturity to describe the changes in fat-free body composition during growth based on the content of water, nitrogen, and ash in the fat-free body. He concluded that many species reach a relatively constant fat-free body composition by 4.5% of their lifespan. Moulton (54) extended this observation to man and estimated that chemical maturity is reached by the age of 3 or 4 years. This concept has been fundamental to investigations into the study of body composition in children and youth for the past 50 years. As a result, various methods validated on adults have been applied to children, assuming the child to be chemically mature. Because children pass through puberty only after a long delayed childhood growth phase as compared to nonprimate mammals, there is reason to question the extent of chemical maturity in the prepubescent child and to reexamine the literature for evidence of chemical immaturity.

TECHNIQUES FOR ASSESSING
BODY COMPOSITION IN CHILDREN

Assuming the young child is chemically mature, that is, the composition of the fat-free body closely approaches that of the adult, several methods have been used to estimate the body composition of children. The methods most often investigated include densitometry, hydrometry, gamma-ray spectrometry, and anthropometry, and these methods have been reviewed for their use in human body composition research by several authors (4,7,24,44,45). The assumptions for use of these methods in children are briefly reviewed here.

Densitometry

Body density in children and adults can be measured by techniques such as underwater weighing, determination of body volume using helium dilution, and water displacement. The most popular method by far, however, is the underwater weighing technique with correction for pulmonary residual volume (11).

Whole body density is a function of the densities of the various body components and the proportion each component occupies with respect to the whole body mass (36). The fact that the density of fat is substantially less than that for other body constituents has led to the development of equations for estimating body fat and fat-free body from body density. Compartmentalizing the body into fat and fat-free parts, however, requires the following basic assumptions: (a) the densities of the two compartments are known and additive; (b) the densities of the fat-free body components, including water, mineral, and protein, are relatively constant from individual to individual; (c) the proportion of each fat-free body component with respect to the total fat-free body is relatively constant from individual to individual; and (d) the individual being assessed differs from a "standard reference individual," upon which a given equation is based, only in the amount of depot fat possessed (10,69). From the first three assumptions (a, b, and c), Siri (69) has derived the following relation between fat content (f, fat as a fraction of body weight) and body density (D) assuming the density of fat is .900 gm/cc and the density of the fat-free body is 1.100 gm/cc:

$$f = \frac{4.95}{D} - 4.50 \qquad \text{(Equation \#1)}$$

From assumptions a, b, and d above, Brozek et al. (10) proposed the following equation:

$$f = \frac{4.570}{D} - 4.142 \qquad \text{(Equation \#2)}$$

Similar values for fat are found from either approach (10); however, neither may be applicable to children since the density of the fat-free body may be significantly less than 1.100 gm/cc. For example, the fat-free body density in an 8-year-old child may be 1.085 gm/cc, as will be proposed later in this chapter. Following Siri's approach using the general equation of Brozek (10) to develop the relation of fatness to density, we have:

$$f = \frac{1}{D} \left(\frac{d_1 d_0}{d_0 - d_1} \right) - \frac{d_1}{d_0 - d_1} \qquad \text{(Equation \#3)}$$

Substituting for $d_1 = .900$ gm/cc (density of fat) and $d_0 = 1.085$ gm/cc (density of fat-free body), we have:

$$f = \frac{5.28}{D} - 4.86$$ (Equation #4)

For a child with a density of 1.050 gm/cc using the adult equation (#1) of Siri (69), a fat content of 21.4% is estimated; however, using the above equation (#4) a fat content of 16.9% is computed. Thus, the estimated fat content may be considerably overestimated in the young child and is clearly dependent upon the actual density of the fat-free body.

Hydrometry

The use of total body water to estimate body composition in terms of fat and fat-free body is based on the assumption that the fat-free body has a relatively constant water content with negligible water associated with the fat stored in adipose tissue. Total body water (TBW) is measured by application of the dilution principle (36). A variety of tracer substances have been used to measure TBW, including antipyrine (22,73) deuterium oxide (18,67) tritium oxide (15,59), and ethanol (39) as well as urea, thiourea, sulfanilamide, and potassium as reported by Pace et al. (59). Each tracer has its advantages and disadvantages; however, most of the body water determinations reported in the literature are based on antipyrine, deuterium oxide, and tritium oxide dilution.

Deuterium oxide appears to be the preferred tracer for use with children since it is not radioactive as is tritium oxide, nor is it metabolized or bound with protein as is antipyrine (67). However, the deuterium and tritium body water spaces may be from 0.5% to 2% larger than the true TBW since these hydrogen isotopes readily exchange with hydrogen in organic compounds of the body (39). The water content of the fat-free body has been proposed to be 73.2% (60) based on data from six species of mammals, 73.7% for the reference body (10), between 69 to 74% (53), and 71.8% of the fat-free body based on adult males (58). Total body water divided by approximately 0.73 is often used to predict the fat-free body weight, with fat calculated by the difference between weight and fat-free body weight. Thus, a 7-year-old child with 15 liters of body water (57) and weighing 23.2 kg would have 20.5 kg of fat-free body weight or 11% fat, assuming a fat-free body water content of 73%. On the other hand, if the water content of the fat-free body is actually higher than assumed, for example 77%, then the fat-free body weight would be 19.5 kg and the percent of body fat content would be 16%. Use of the adult hydrometric model for children then leads to an underestimation of relative body fatness.

Densitometry and Hydrometry

Siri (68,69) has suggested that variability in water content of the fat-free body may be the largest source of variation in the density of the fat-free body of adults. Bakker and Struikenkamp (3) and Lohman (42) further estimated the variability in density associated with water variability in adults. Siri (69) proposed the following equation when both body density (D) and body water (w), expressed as a percent of body weight, were known in the same subjects.

$$f = \frac{2.118}{D} - .78w - 1.354 \qquad \text{(Equation \#5)}$$

Using this approach, then, a 7-year-old child with a density of 1.050 gm/cc and a water content of 65% body weight would have an estimated fat content of 15.6%.

Gamma-Ray Spectrometry

Body potassium can be measured by assessing the naturally occurring 40_K (gamma-ray spectrometry) using a whole body counter or by isotope dilution using 40_K. For either method the potassium content of the body can be calculated and body composition estimates can be made. Thus, measurement of the potassium content of the human body serves as an index of the fat-free body mass in much the same way as measurement of body water. Again, the primary assumption is that the fat-free body has a constant potassium content. Forbes and Hursh (26) proposed a potassium content of 2.66 gm/kg fat-free body of 68.1 mEq, based on four human adult cadavers for which a tissue chemical analysis was conducted. This value has been widely accepted by many investigators for children and adults. More recently the potassium content of adult females has been found to be 10% less than for males, or about 2.4 gm/kg. In children, 2.66 gm/kg FFB has been used by most investigators; however, lower values may be more appropriate, as indicated later in this chapter.

For a 7-year-old child with total body potassium mass of 63 gms, a fat-free body mass of 24 kg would be predicted assuming 2.66 gm/kg. For a child weighing 30 kg, 20% fat would be estimated. If a 2.40 gm/kg of fat-free body were assumed, the fat content would then be 12%.

Anthropometry

Measurement of skinfold thicknesses, body circumferences, and widths have received widespread use as a method to estimate body composition in children and adults. To validate the use of anthropometry as an index of body composition, body fat is not measured directly but rather through indirect methods such as densitometry, hydrometry, or gamma-ray spectrometry. These methods are assumed to be valid for the sample under study. Many multiple regression equations using anthropometric dimensions have been developed for various populations. Adult an-thropometric equations overestimate the body density of children (43), and equations developed on children may overestimate the body fatness since they are based on the criterion methods densitometry, hydrometry, and gamma-ray spectrometry, which need further validation for this young population before they can be applied for routine measurement of body composition.

WATER CONTENT OF THE FAT-FREE BODY

The water content of the adult human body is approximately 60% of the body weight but may vary greatly (Table 2-1) depending on body fatness and gender (36,51). However, due to a lack of information, the water content of the growing child, particularly from 6 to 18 years of age, has not been adequately described. The extent to which body water changes, especially as a fraction of fat-free body during pre- and postpubescent growth and development and during the remaining aging process, is not well established. Friis-Hansen (29) has suggested that the water content expressed relative to body weight (%TBW) decreases from 78% at birth to about 60% at 1 year, approximating the relative adult water content in both males and females (Table 2-2). Further, the distribution of the total body water appears to change during growth with a general trend toward a relative reduction in the extracellular water and an increase in the in-tracellular water (Table 2-2). Friis-Hansen (29) also observed that %TBW increases slightly from 1 to 3 years with respect to the adult values achieved at 1 year and then declines slowly until adult values are again achieved. Moulton (54) has estimated chemical maturity for body water and solids to be established at age 3 to 4 years. These results, however, were based on chemical analysis of fetuses, infants, and adults, but not of children or adolescents (Figure 2-1).

Forbes (24) cites data from the literature which suggest that mature water content is reached in childhood, but does not specify the age. There is also evidence that the %TBW may decline slightly prior to puberty in males due to increased fat storage. Heald et al. (30) found that %TBW increased from 12 to 16 years in males, at which time adult values are reached, suggesting that adult body water is not reached prior to age 16 in males. Data within this age span for females presented by Young et al. (83) show a reverse trend to that of males, with %TBW generally decreasing, possibly due to increased accumulation of fat. Although these estimates are based on limited data, the suggestion that

Table 2-1

Age Trends Percent of Total Body Water and the Water Content of the Fat-Free Body[1]

Source	Age	N	%TBW	TBW/FFW[2]
Male Children				
Novak (57)	6-7	39	65.4[D]	.769
Heald et al. (30)	12	7	60.9	.755
	13	6	61.6[D]	.748
	14	9	62.4[D]	.743
	15	9	63.1[D]	.736
	16	7	63.8[D]	.731
	17	6	64.5[D]	.726
	18	1	65.1[D]	.719
Female Children				
Novak (57)	6-7	25	61.7[D]	.763
Young et al. (83)	9-10	20	63.0[A]	.770
	11	13	56.4[A]	.802
	12	21	59.8[A]	.775
	13	13	61.0[A]	.777
	14	15	59.7[A]	.764
	15	9	52.9[A]	.714
	16	12	54.6[A]	.737
	Pre-menstr.	56	61.0	.775
	Post-menstr.	46	56.3	.751
Adults				
Bolleau et al. (6)				
Normal	18	15	62.5[D]	.735
Obese	18	8	45.4[D]	.738
Pascale et al. (64)				
Lean	19	12	62.7[D]	.708
Buskirk & Taylor (12)	22	41	54.2[A]	.690
Loeppky et al. (39)	20-30	13	60.9[T]	.738
	30-40	19	61.9[T]	.741
Young et al. (83)	16-30	94	51.7[A]	.729
	30-40	26	49.3[A]	.713
Lesser et al. (38)	19-25	3	56.2[T]	.711[C]

[1]Density (D_b) for this study was computed from skinfolds using equation of Pařizkova (61).

$$\%FFW = 1 - [2.118/D_b - .78\,(\tfrac{TBW}{BW}) - 1.354]\,100$$

[2]%FFW was computed from mean body density and total body water data reported for each study according to equation of Siri (69).

[A]TBW determined by antipyrine.

[D]TBW determined by deuterium oxide.

[T]TBW determined by tritium oxide.

Table 2.2

Mean Values of Total Body Water, Extracellular Water and Intracellular Water Expressed as a Percentage of Body Weight as Reported by Friis-Hansen (29)

Age of subjects	%TBW	(N)	%ECW	(N)	%ICW	(N)
0-1 day	78.4	(21)[1]	44.5	(10)	33.9	(10)
1-30 days	74.0	(9)	39.7	(4)	31.8	(4)
1-3 months	72.3	(7)	32.2	(3)	43.3	(3)
3-6 months	70.1	(5)	30.1	(3)	42.1	(3)
6-12 months	60.4	(8)	27.4	(5)	35.2	(5)
1-2 years	58.7	(5)	25.6	(4)	33.6	(2)
2-3 years	63.5	(9)	26.7	(8)	38.3	(6)
3-5 years	62.2	(6)	21.4	(2)	45.7	(2)
5-10 years	61.5	(4)	22.0	(13)	42.3	(10)
10-15 years	57.3	(13)	18.7	(5)	46.7	(1)

[1]Numbers in parentheses indicate the number of subjects measured.

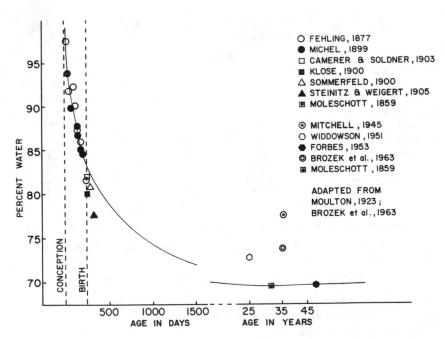

Figure 2-1. Relationship between age and the water content of the fat-free body in man. Adapted from Moulton (54) and Brozek et al. (10).

extra- and intracellular solids which osmotically control water content are established at adult levels in the first 4 years of life needs further scrutiny.

The most complete data across the childhood years have been reported by Heald et al. (30) and Young et al. (83), who measured boys ages 12 to 18 years and girls ages 9 to 17 years, respectively. By recalculating the data of Heald et al. (30), it can be observed that the water content of the fat-free body decreases rather uniformly in boys over the age span studied at the rate of approximately 0.6% per year from 75.8% to 71.9% (Figure 2-2). These calculations are based on both water and density to estimate fat content. Using Siri's (69) method (Equation #5), the fat content of 12-year-old children in the Heald sample would be 19.3%, and thus the water content of the fat-free body would be 75.8% (60.9/80.7).

Calculations of the fat-free body water content (Table 2-1) from data of Young et al. (83) show a decrease in water content after menarche (77.5% before and 75.1% after) and suggest that the adult level may not be reached until 15 years of age. As mentioned earlier, the changes in hydration of the fat-free body during growth and development contradict the assumption of constancy of the fat-free body. Variability in the water content of the fat-free body during growth and development has an important effect on the estimation of body composition (% fat) from body density measurements since the variation in water content of the fat-free body appears to exert the greatest influence on variation in the density of the fat-free body (42).

In summary, the water content of the fat-free body in both prepubescent boys and girls may be higher than the 71 to 73% typically found in adults (Figure 2-2). During the pubescent and postpubescent period the

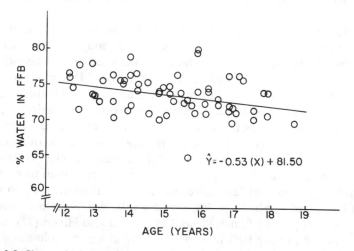

Figure 2-2. Changes in the water content of the fat-free body in relation to the age of young males 12-18 years. Data from Heald et al. (30).

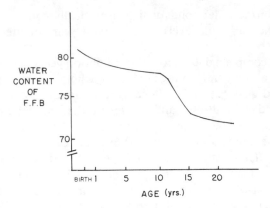

Figure 2-3. Hypothetical changes in the water content of the fat-free body during growth and development.

water content of the fat-free body appears to decrease from 77% to 72%, based on changes estimated from body water and body density. A hypothetical developmental curve is presented in Figure 2-3 which suggests possible changes in the water content of the fat-free body as a function of age. The use of body water by itself to estimate body composition may result in underestimating the percent of fat in children if the adult value of 72-73% (water content of fat-free body) is used. Further research into the water content of the fat-free body in pre- and postpubescent children is needed to substantiate the findings of Heald et al. (30) and Young et al. (83).

BONE MINERAL CONTENT OF THE FAT-FREE BODY

Variation in the bone mineral content of the body is the second major source of variation in the density of the fat-free body in the mature adult (3,42,69). Moulton (54) summarized the work of several investigators and found the ash content of the fat-free body of the infant to be between 3 and 4% as compared to 9% for the adult male (Figure 2-4). Data from direct analysis of human cadavers have been summarized by Keys and Brozek (36). For the ash content of the body, data are given in Table 2-3 from five cadavers, and Keys and Brozek (36) conclude that man has an ash content of the fat-free body of 7.2%. Brozek et al. (10) estimated the mineral content of the fat-free body in reference man to be 6.8%. Women appear to have less dense skeletal tissue than men, as do whites when compared to blacks (9,76). Based on the difference between bone densities in males and females found by Trotter and Hixon (77), women would appear to have 10% less bone mineral in a given volume of bone. This would decrease the density of the fat-free body to 1.095 gm/cc (Table 2-4).

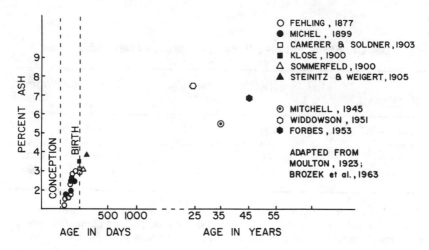

Figure 2-4. Relationship between age and the ash content of the fat-free body in man. Adapted from Moulton (54) and Brozek et al. (10).

Table 2-3

Ash Content of the Fat-Free Body in Five Adult Cadavers[1]

Age	Sex	Height (cm)	Weight (kg)	Ash of Body (%)	Ash of Fat-Free Body (%)
42	F	169	45.1	7.6	9.9
46	M	168.5	53.8	5.4	6.7
35	M	183	70.6	4.8	5.5
25	M	170	71.8	7.5	8.8
48	M	—	63.8	4.9	5.0
M				6.0	7.2

[1]Keys & Brozek (36)

Moulton's (54) concept of chemical maturity was revised by Spray and Widdowson (74), who showed that the time of chemical maturity varies with the constituent. For instance, in the rat it has been shown that the potassium concentration rises rapidly in the fat-free body during the first 30 days of postnatal development and then remains about the same for at least the next 320 days, whereas calcium concentration increases for 100 days after birth before leveling off. Forbes (24) suggests that children may reach a calcium content of 21 gm per kg of fat-free body, a value close to the adult value. However, Forbes (24) also describes the total body calcium growth curve for males and females and shows an ac-

Table 2-4

Density of the Fat-Free Body in Reference Man and Woman

Constituent	Reference Man[1] %	Density	Reference Woman[1] %	Density
Water	.738	.99371	.744	.99371
Protein	.194	1.34	.195	1.34
Mineral	.068	3.038	.061	3.038
Fat-free body		1.100		1.095

[1]Densities and proportions of body constituents for reference man from Brozek et al. (10). For reference woman mineral was decreased 10% as compared to reference man, and water and protein content proportionately increased.

celerated growth of calcium from the pre- to postpubescent years. This accelerated growth may not be proportional to the fat-free body growth. For instance, the total body calcium doubles in boys from 12 to 18 years of age (17) while body weight increases by a factor of 1.7.

Trotter and Hixon (77), in an extensive study of changes in the weight, density, and percent ash weight of human skeletons from an early fetal period through childhood, adulthood, and old age, found some increases in ash content of certain bones from birth to 22 years of age. In general, Trotter and Hixon found that the densities of the bones tested increased with age to adulthood. Gender differences, with male bones being heavier than female bones, are more marked than race differences, with bones of blacks being heavier than those of whites.

A variety of approaches are available for estimating either dry, fat-free skeletal mass or total bone mineral. Anthropometry (2,46), radiographic densitometry (52,75,76), direct photon absorptiometry (47,78), and total body neutron activation (55) have been used.

With the development of photon absorptiometry, bone mineral content (gm/cm) of a 1-cm cross-section and bone width of various bones can be measured *in vivo* in children and adults (13,14). This method, by utilizing a photon source of monoenergetic, low energy gamma rays (^{125}I), passes the radioactive source at a uniform speed across the bone, and the transmitted radiation is measured with a collimated NaI crystal detector.

Data obtained by Mazess and Cameron (49) on 245 children and adults are summarized for the distal third of the radius for selected ages in Table 2-5. Bone mineral (gm/cm) more than doubles between 8 years of age and the adult value, which appears to reach its peak somewhere between 20 and 40 years of age. Bone width increases 44% in boys and 33% in girls over the same age range. Adjusting the bone mineral content

Table 2-5

Bone Mineral Content and Width of the Distal Third of Radius of Children, Youth, and Adults of Selected Age[1]

Radius	Age (years)						
	8	11	14	17	20-29	30-39	40-49
Bone mineral (gm/cm)							
Male	.56	.70	.90	1.20	1.31	1.32	1.30
Female	.48	.65	.84	.89	.95	1.00	.98
Bone width (cm)							
Male	1.03	1.15	1.30	1.45	1.48	1.48	1.48
Female	.92	1.07	1.18	1.22	1.23	1.30	1.30
Bone mineral (gm/cm²)							
Male	.55	.61	.69	.83	.89	.90	.88
Female	.52	.61	.71	.73	.77	.77	.76
Number of subjects/group	56	65	63	61	231	101	106

[1]Mazess & Cameron (48)

(gm/cm) for differences in bone width shows a marked increase from childhood to adulthood in bone mineral per cm² (62% increase in males and 48% increase in females). Similar results have been found by Mazess and Mather (50) in the Alaskan Eskimo children, and by Christiansen et al. (17) in Danish children. Because estimates of the depth of bone cannot be made by most photon absorptiometric instruments, bone density (gm/cm³) cannot be computed. Thus, changes in bone density with age are not well documented under the present development of this methodology, with the exception of a study by Klemm, Banzer, and Schneider (37).

In the study by Klemm et al. (37), bone density has been measured in children for the os calcis bone. This technique has been described by Schneider and Banzer (66). It involves modification of the photon absorptiometric method to include several radiographs in the plane of measurement enabling an estimate of the volume of cross-section of bone assayed for mineral by the absorptiometric method. Bone mineral content and density were measured in 66 boys ages 3 to 16 years and in 71 girls ages 3 to 20 years. While bone mineral content of the os calcis at the age of 6 years had only reached 33% of the adult value, the bone density (g/cm³) was found to be 67% of the adult value. By the age of 15, girls were found to have reached 90% of their adult density; boys at 15 had reached only 80% of their adult bone density. From the results of Klemm et al. (37), we have developed the following table for bone density changes in children and youth expressed as a percent of a standard for normal adults (Table 2-6).

Table 2-6

**Bone Density Expressed as a Percent
of an Adult Standard for the Oscalcis[1]**

			Age			
Sex	5-6	7-8	11-12	15	20	25
Males	62	68	73	80	90	100
Females	62	68	80	90	90	100

[1]Data estimated from Figure 1 of Klemm et al. (37).

Mazess and Cameron (48) studied skeletal growth in 322 white children ages 6 to 14 years, measuring bone mineral by photon absorptiometry and skeletal age by hand-wrist radiographs. They found skeletal age to be a poor predictor of bone mineral content which did not decrease the predictive error substantially more than chronological age. Partial correlations of both age and skeletal age with bone mineral content were less than $r = 0.10$ when body size was held constant. They conclude that skeletal age relates primarily to body size and not to skeletal status as reflected in bone mineral content. Thus, it seems necessary to measure bone mineral content directly rather than through association with skeletal maturity.

In summary, the bone mineral content of the fat-free body in prepubescent boys and girls appears to be less than the 7% adult value. Evidence of a lower mineral content comes from research showing lower bone densities and smaller bone size and mineral content. The exact bone mineral content of the fat-free body and its change with age has not yet been established. The theoretical changes in the bone mineral content of the fat-free body as a function of age and gender are illustrated in Figure 2-5. Research is needed to establish the relative change in bone mineral content of the fat-free body in growing children.

CHANGES IN POTASSIUM CONTENT
OF THE FAT-FREE BODY

The potassium content of the fat-free body has been found to be quite constant in the adult animal and to reach its upper limit after puberty in several animal species (26). Almost all potassium is intracellular and over 70% is found in the muscle and viscera. Additional amounts are found in the bone and cartilage, with less than 6% found in adipose tissue. Consequently, almost all potassium is contained within the fat-free body with

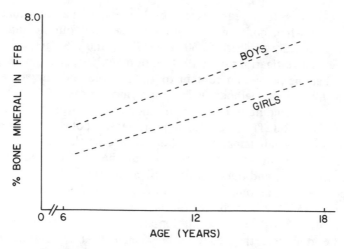

Figure 2-5. Hypothetical changes in the bone mineral content of the fat-free body as a function of sex and age during growth and development.

the skeletal muscle containing the most potassium (Table 2-7). In animals, Lohman (40) estimated the biological variation of potassium to be less than 4% on a fat-free basis.

Based on the assumption that the potassium content of the fat-free body is constant in humans as well as animals, Forbes, Gallup, and Hursh (25) proposed a quantitative relation between body potassium and

Table 2-7

Potassium Distribution in Two Cadavers as Determined by Direct Chemical Analysis

Tissue	K Content (gm/kg)	K Mass (gm)	Proportion of Body K (%)
Muscle	3.41	96.5	61.6
Skeleton	1.32	12.7	8.1
Adipose	2.54	9.1	5.8
Skin	1.93	7.8	5.0
Nerve	3.15	5.5	3.5
Lungs	2.54	5.3	3.4
Liver	2.73	4.5	2.9
GI	1.41	1.9	1.2
Heart	2.30	0.8	0.5
Kidney	2.05	0.6	0.4
Remainder	2.28	11.9	7.6

Forbes & Lewis (27)

fat-free body mass (referred to as lean body mass) with a potassium content of the fat-free body of 2.66 gm/kg based on four human adult cadavers chemically analyzed (2.60, 2.60, 2.61, and 2.85 gm/kg). Data from various investigations since 1961 on humans have been summarized to show that the potassium content of the fat-free body in women, as estimated by various methods, is less than that for men (5,28). A summary of selected findings grouped by method of measuring fat-free body is given in Table 2-8. The results all support a lower potassium content of fat-free body in adult females. In addition, Womersley et al. (82) have found differences in potassium content of the fat-free body among athletic, sedentary, and obese subjects of both sexes.

For children, the amount of potassium in the fat-free body is not well documented. While it is fairly well established that the potassium content of the fat-free body of the adult female is between 90 and 95% of that of the adult male, the difference between male and female prepubescent children is less apparent.

Forbes (23,24), in describing the growth of children in fat and fat-free body between 8 and 29 years of age based on [40]K estimates, points out that little data are found in the literature on the change in the potassium content of the fat-free body in children. His fat-free estimates assume the potassium content of the fat-free body is 2.66 gm/kg for boys through the age range and a decreasing potassium content of the fat-free body in

Table 2-8

Potassium Content of Fat-Free Body Mass in Males and Females by Method and Investigator

Method of Measuring FFB/ Investigator	Males			Females			Male/ Female Ratio of K/FFB
	Age	N	K/FFB	Age	N	K/FFB	
FFB from height and weight							
Womersley et al. (81)	17-30	10	2.59	17-30	10	2.28	.88
Boddy et al. (5)	20-77	49	2.53	20-77	54	2.22	.88
FFB from anthropometry							
Womersley et al. (81)	17-30	10	2.63	17-30	10	2.45	.93
Pierson et al. (65)	21-50	182	2.65	21-50	308	2.26	.85
FFB from body water							
Delwaide (20)	20	53	2.45	20	59	2.22	.91
Allen et al. (1)	16-51	28	2.56	16-51	10	2.29	.89
FFB from body density							
Womersley et al. (81)	17-30	10	2.56	17-30	10	2.34	.91
Womersley et al. (81)	17-30	12	2.62	17-32	12	2.35	.90

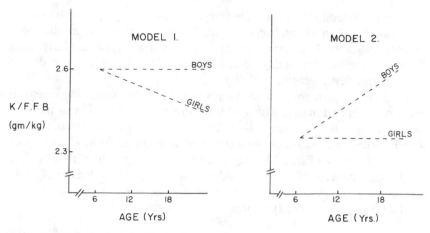

Figure 2-6. Hypothetical changes in the potassium content of the fat-free body as a function of sex and age during growth and development.

girls as follows: 8 to 12 years, 2.66 gm/kg; 13 to 15, 2.61 gm/kg; 16 to 18, 2.53 gm/kg; and 2.50 gm/kg for the adult female (Figure 2-6, Model 1).

Recently, Slaughter, Lohman, and Boileau (72) discussed the difficulty of determining the potassium content of the fat-free body from the previous research. They concluded that the potassium content may range from 2.5 to 2.7 gm/kg FFB in young boys and girls based on the data of Allen, Anderson, and Langham (1), Cheek (16), and Cureton, Boileau, and Lohman (19). A second hypothetical model for describing the change in potassium content in the fat-free body was proposed (72). The authors suggested that boys and girls have comparable amounts of potassium per unit of fat-free body before puberty and somewhat less than 2.66 gm/kg. After puberty the potassium mass increases greatly in males as compared to females. This increase is partly associated with an increase in the proportion of muscle in the fat-free body of boys, and causes the potassium content of the fat-free body to increase to the adult male value of 2.66 gm/kg (Figure 2-6, Model 2). Further studies are needed to determine the potassium content of the fat-free body of prepubescent children before growth and development of the fat-free body can be accurately assessed using ⁴⁰K methodology.

CHANGES IN DENSITY OF THE FAT-FREE BODY

The assumption that the density of the fat-free body is constant throughout growth and development is subject to question in light of the possible changes within this component, particularly with respect to body water and bone mineral content. Both of these constituents have densities markedly different from the fat-free body as a whole, that is, water, 0.994 gm/cc at 36°C and bone mineral 3.317 gm/cc. Therefore they contribute substantially to change in fat-free body density, particularly when both change systematically to increase fat-free body density during growth and development.

If the water content decreases with age, then the remaining constituents as a proportion of the fat-free body increase, resulting in an increase in the fat-free body density (d_{ffb}). Theoretical changes as related to age can be calculated assuming the water content changes from 77 to 72% of the fat-free body (Table 2-9). For example, a 12-year-old with a fat-free body water content of 75.1% would have a fat-free body density of 1.082 gm/cc, assuming a density of the dry fat-free body (protein and mineral) of 1.48 gm/cc and density of water of .9937 gm/cc. Thus:

$$\frac{1}{d_{ffb}} = \frac{.751}{.9937} + \frac{.249}{1.48}$$

$$d_{ffb} = 1.082 \text{ gm/cc} \qquad \text{(Equation \#6)}$$

Similarly, it can be shown that an increase in the bone mineral content of the fat-free body also results in an increase in the fat-free body density. From both decreases in body water and increases in bone mineral, one can calculate the theoretical changes in fat-free body density with age.

Table 2-9

Change in Body Density From an Increase in Water and Decrease in Body Mineral Content

Age Group	Fat-Free Body		Body (%)				Theoretical Density[3] (gm/cc)
	Water[1]	Mineral[2]	Fat	Water	Mineral	Protein	
Men (age 20-29)	72	6.8	12	64	6.1	17.9	1.076
Boys (age 8-10)	77	4.6	12	69	4.1	14.9	1.051

[1]Body water content of the fat-free body of 8- to 10-year-old boys estimated from the data of Heald et al. (30) and Young et al. (83).

[2]Mineral content of the fat-free body of children estimated to be 67% of the adult value of Klemm et al. (37).

[3]Body density calculated from the fat, water, mineral, and protein content of young men and boys assuming the following densities for each component: fat, .9007 gm/cc; water, .9937 gm/cc; mineral, 3.317 gm/cc; and protein, 1.34 gm/cc.

Furthermore, one can compare the overall density of the body in prepubescent children versus the adult, holding body fat constant. The results of these calculations are given in Table 2-9. In the following equation the density of the body (D) can be determined by using the densities of its parts at 36°C in the denominator: that is, the density of fat (df = .9007 gm/cc), of water (dw = .9937 gm/cc), of mineral (dm = 3.317 gm/cc), and of protein (dp = 1.34 gm/cc); and the fraction of mass of each part of the whole in the numerators, that is, fat content of body (f), water content (w), mineral content (m), and protein content (p).

$$\frac{1}{D} = \frac{f}{df} + \frac{w}{dw} + \frac{m}{dm} + \frac{p}{dp} \qquad \text{(Equation \#7)}$$

For the adult fat-free body, that is, 72% water and 6.8% bone mineral in the fat-free body, and a fat content of 12%, the water, mineral, and protein content of the body can be calculated by difference: w = .64, m = .061, p = .179 (Table 2-9). For young men then, a fat content of 12% is equivalent to a density of 1.076 gm/cc. On the other hand, for 8- to 10-year-old boys with 12% fat the following estimation is made (Equation #8) based on water, mineral, and protein contents of 69%, 4.1%, and 14.9%, respectively.

$$\frac{1}{D} = \frac{.12}{.9007} + \frac{.690}{.9937} + \frac{.041}{3.317} + \frac{.149}{1.34} = .9512$$

$$D = 1.051 \text{ gm/cc} \qquad \text{(Equation \#8)}$$

Thus, the differences in the density of the fat-free body between children and adults, as hypothetically demonstrated in the above examples, clearly suggests that serious underestimation of body density result for the child when subjected to the adult model due to significant differences between children and adults in the composition of the fat-free body.

Various researchers have found similar increases in the overall body density in males from prepubescence to postpubescence. These increases are summarized in Table 2-10. For females, slight decreases are found in density. Also summarized is the weighted mean density of children between 8 and 11 years of age for nine investigations for boys (n = 463) and five for girls (n = 204). These increases in body density for males are interpreted as a decline in fat content and increase in fat-free body size and proportion. The extent to which changes in fat-free body development affect body density apart from fatness may influence our understanding of growth changes during puberty. Present estimates, such as those of Pařizkova (62), may overestimate the actual growth velocity of the fat-free body, especially for boys.

Table 2-10

Body Density Changes With Age

Reference	Age Range (yrs.)	Body Density Changes
Males		
Hunt & Heald (31)	12 to 17	1.047 to 1.076
Novak (56)	13.5 to 17.5	1.065 to 1.074
Pařizkova (62)	7.5 to 16.5	1.061 to 1.073
Pařizkova (63)	10.7 to 17.7	1.057 to 1.076
M density of 9 investigations	7 to 11	1.054
Females		
Young et al. (83)	9.5 to 16	1.041 to 1.035
Pařizkova (62)	8.5 to 17.6	1.048 to 1.044
M density of 5 investigations	7 to 11	1.040

ANTHROPOMETRY AND BODY FAT ESTIMATES IN CHILDREN

The use of skinfolds, circumferences, and skeletal widths are frequently applied in the adult population as a field method for body fatness. Equations for prediction of body composition from anthropometric dimensions are characterized by standard errors of prediction of between 3 and 5% fat. For children, anthropometric dimensions are also useful in estimating percent fat, with a standard error of estimate only slightly larger than in adults (42). It has been observed, however, that prediction equations applicable to adults do not apply to children (43). The change in the relationship between anthropometric dimensions and body fatness as estimated from body density appears to take place between 8 and 15 years of age. Thus, the interpretation of skinfold data (triceps and subscapular) collected as part of the National Health Survey on children from 6 to 17 years of age (Table 2-11) in terms of total body fatness cannot be made at the present time.

That the adult equations employing skinfolds and density cannot be used with children is illustrated from the data of Durnin and Rahaman (21) on 48 boys ages 12.7 to 15.7 and 38 girls ages 13.2 to 16.4, in comparison to adult groups ages 18 to 34 years. For the sum of four skinfolds of 40 mm, corresponding densities of 1.060, 1.050, 1.043, and 1.042 gm/cc were found for boys, men, girls, and women, respectively. By using Sloan's equations, derived from college men and women (70,71), and applying them to children using the mean thigh and subscapular skinfold sites to predict body density for boys (70) and the mean of suprailiac and triceps sites for girls (71), the inapplicability of adult equations can also be shown. These results are summarized in Table 2-12. They show that in

Table 2-11

Median Values for Sum of Triceps and Subscapular Skinfolds in Children and Youth

	Age (yrs.)											
Sex	6	7	8	9	10	11	12	13	14	15	16	17
	Median Sum of Skinfolds (mm)											
Males	12	12	13	14	14	16	15	15	14	15	15	16
Females	14	15	16	17	18	19	19	20	24	25	25	27

Based on data from Johnston, Hamill, & Lemeshow (32,33).

Table 2-12

Predicted Density in Children, Youth, and Adults From Adult Skinfold Equations

Age (Investigator)	Males		Females	
	Predicted Density[1]	Actual Density[2]	Predicted Density[3]	Actual Density[2]
Children				
9-12, Pařizkova (61)	1.072	1.048	1.048	1.040
8-11, Boileau et al. (8)	1.072	1.050	1.053	1.035
Nonmenarche, Young et al. (83)			1.056	1.037
Youth				
13-16, Pařizkova (61)	1.076	1.060	1.049	1.047
Menarche, Young et al. (83)	—	—	1.051	1.037
17, Katch & Michael (35)	1.070	1.074	—	—
Adults				
Wilmore & Behnke (79,80)	1.066	1.066	1.051	1.041
Lohman et al. (41)	1.068	1.065	1.046	1.041
Katch & McArdle (34)	1.065	1.065	1.036	1.039

[1]Density predicted from Sloan's (70) equation using thigh and subscapular skinfolds derived from 50 male students ages 18 to 26.

[2]Density as measured from underwater weighing of the subject.

[3]Density predicted from Sloan et al.'s (71) equation using suprailiac and triceps skinfolds derived from 50 female students ages 17 to 25.

children 8 to 12 years of age, body density is overestimated by about .023 gm/cc in boys (10% fat underestimation; predicted value 12%, observed value 22%) and .01 gm/cc in girls. For youths 13 to 16 years of age, the overestimation of density is somewhat less in boys than in girls. For adults, Sloan's equations have been studied extensively in a number of cross-validation studies and found to be one of the most valid equations yet derived for the college-age male population (42). In several cross-validation studies in men and women, mean predicted values are close to the density values measured, particularly for men (Table 2-12).

Finally, using the data of Young et al. (83), the relationship between the sum of 12 skinfolds and body density was calculated for prepubescent, pubescent, and postpubescent girls. The predicted densities corresponding to the mean skinfold thickness of the entire sample were 1.033 gm/cc for the prepubescent group, 1.036 gm/cc for the pubescent group, and 1.041 gm/cc for the postpubescent group. Thus, the body density increases with maturation for a given skinfold in both girls and boys. Further research is needed before anthropometric dimensions can be used to estimate body composition in children. For now, use of equations derived from underwater weighing of children leads to an overestimation of fatness while use of adult equations on children appears to underestimate fatness (43).

FAT-FREE COMPOSITION OF PREPUBESCENT CHILDREN AND IMPLICATIONS FOR BODY COMPOSITION ESTIMATES

Evidence has been presented to indicate that the composition of the fat-free body in prepubescent children may differ significantly from the adult. The water, bone mineral, and potassium content may all differ, with prepubescent children having a higher water content and lower bone mineral and potassium contents. The fat-free body density would also be lower in children. Further research is needed to substantiate the above hypothesis and to determine when children become chemically mature. Meanwhile, caution should be placed on estimates of body composition in children from the conventional methods. It appears that the methods are reliable; however, body fat may be overestimated by using adult constants based on body density and body potassium and underestimated for body water.

From body density one can estimate the fat-free body density of an 8-year-old boy assuming a mineral content of 4.6%, a water content of 77%, and a protein content of 18.4%. The fat-free density would be 1.085 gm/cc. Assuming this density is more appropriate for children, one can derive the following formula for estimation of percent fat by application of Equation #3. If:

ADULT (F.F.B DENSITY =1.10 gm/cc)		CHILDREN (F.F.B DENSITY=1.085gm/cc)	
DENSITY	% FAT	DENSITY	% FAT
1.10	0		
1.09	4.1		
		1.085	0
1.08	8.3	1.08	2.2
1.07	12.6	1.07	6.8
1.06	17.0	1.06	11.4
1.05	21.4	1.05	16.2
1.04	26.0	1.04	21.0
1.03	30.6	1.03	25.9
1.02	35.3	1.02	31.0
1.01	40.1	1.01	36.1
1.00	45.0	1.00	41.3

Figure 2-7. Body density and relative fatness in adults and children when using different assumed densities of the fat-free body.

$$f = \frac{1}{D} \left(\frac{d_1 d_0}{d_0 - d_1} \right) - \frac{d_1}{d_0 - d_1} \qquad \text{(Equation #3)}$$

Then:

$$\% \text{ fat} = \frac{1}{D} \left(\frac{0.900 \quad 1.085}{1.085 - .900} \right) - \frac{.900}{1.085 - .900} \qquad \text{(Equation #9)}$$

Figure 2-7 illustrates the results of using the Siri (69) equation compared with the newly derived Equation (#4) which is believed to be more appropriate for children.

$$f = \frac{5.28}{D} - 4.86 \qquad \text{(Equation #4)}$$

SUMMARY

The body fat content of a child is typically estimated from an adult model which assumes that the child's body composition is chemically mature. However, it has been noted that although there are changes in the body density of both males and females during childhood growth and development, the change in density is not due solely to variation in fat. content since significant changes also occur in the fat-free body. Therefore, the concept of chemical maturity has been carefully reviewed with respect to the constancy of the fat-free body. Evidence indicates that prepubescent and adolescent children are not chemically mature and may have a fat-free body density lower than the adult. Specifically, the lower fat-free body density results from a higher water content and lower bone density. Thus, by employing conventional methodological approaches to estimate body composition in children, that is, adult models, estimates of fat and fat-free body may be inaccurate and may lead to biased estimates of body composition and growth in children. Furthermore, anthropometric estimates of body composition are also limited in their accuracy since they are often based on density from underwater weighing and body potassium from gamma-ray spectrometry. Since chemical maturity of the body composition may not be attained until late adolescence, documentation of changes in the composition of the fat-free body as a function of age and maturation is needed. Further research investigating the fat-free body composition of children may bring about a more accurate assessment of the body composition in children.

REFERENCES

1. Allen, T.H., E.C. Anderson, and W.H. Langham. Total body potassium and gross body composition in relation to age. *J. Gerontol.,* 15:348-357, 1960.

2. Allen, T.H., and J.H. Krzywick. "From body water to bone mineral and back." In *Techniques for measuring body composition,* edited by J. Brozek and A. Henschel. Washington: National Academy of Science, 1961.

3. Bakker, H.K., and R.S. Struikenkamp. Biological variability and lean body mass estimates. *Hum. Biol.,* 49:187-202, 1977.

4. Behnke, A.R., and J.H. Wilmore. *Evaluation and regulation of body build and composition.* Englewood Cliffs, NJ: Prentice-Hall, 1974.

5. Boddy, K., P.C. King, J. Womersley, and J.V.G.A. Durnin. Body potassium and fat free mass. *Clin. Sci.,* 44:621-625, 1973.

6. Boileau, R.A., E.R. Buskirk, D.H. Horstman, J. Mendez, and W.C. Nicholas. Body change in obese and lean men during physical conditioning. *Med. Sci. Sports,* 3:183-189, 1971.

7. Boileau, R.A., and T.G. Lohman. The measurement of human physique and its effect on physical performance. *Orthop. Clin. North Amer.,* 8:563-581, 1977.

8. Boileau, R.A., J.H. Wilmore, T.G. Lohman, M.H. Slaughter, W.F. Riner. Estimation of body density from skinfold thicknesses, body circumferences and skeletal widths in boys aged 8 to 11 years: Comparison of two samples. *Hum. Biol.,* 53:575-592, 1981.

9. Brozek, J. "The measurement of body composition." In *Introduc-*

tion to physical anthropology, edited by A. Montogue. Springfield, IL: Thomas, 1960.

10. Brozek, J., F. Grande, J.T. Anderson, and A. Keys. Densitometric analysis of body composition: Revision of some quantitative assumptions. *Ann. NY Acad. Sci.*, 110:113-140, 1963.

11. Buskirk, E.R. "Underwater weighing and body density: A review of procedures." In *Techniques for measuring body composition*, edited by J. Brozek and A. Henschel. Washington: National Academy of Science, 1961.

12. Buskirk, E.R., and H.L. Taylor. Maximal oxygen intake and its relation to body composition with special reference to chronic physical activity and obesity. *J. Appl. Physiol.*, 11:72-78, 1957.

13. Cameron, J.R., R.B. Mazess, and J.A. Sorenson. Precision and accuracy of bone mineral determination by direct photon absorptiometry. *Invest. Radiol.*, 3:141-150, 1968.

14. Cameron, J.R., and J.A. Sorenson. Measurement of bone mineral *in vivo*: An improved method. *Science*, 140:230-232, 1963.

15. Cardus, D., W.G. McTaggart, and C.L. Young. Effect of exercise on determination of total body water by tritium oxide. *J. Appl. Physiol.*, 27:1-3, 1969.

16. Cheek, D.B. *Human growth: Body composition, cell growth, energy and intelligence*. Philadelphia: Lea & Febiger, 1968.

17. Christiansen, C., P. Rodbru, and C.T. Nielsen. Bone mineral content and estimated total body calcium in normal children and adolescents. *Scand. J. Clin. Lab. Invest.*, 35:507-510, 1975.

18. Cook, D.R., W.S. Gualitiere, and S.J. Calla. Body fluid volumes of college athletes and non-athletes. *Med. Sci. Sports*, 1:217-229, 1969.

19. Cureton, K.J., R.A. Boileau, and T.G. Lohman. A comparison of densitometric, potassium 40 and skinfold estimates of body composition. *Hum. Biol.*, 47:321-336, 1975.

20. Delwaide, P.A., and E.J. Crenier. Body potassium as related to lean body mass measured by total water determination and by anthropometric method. *Hum. Biol.*, 45:509-526, 1973.

21. Durnin, J.V.G.A., and M.M. Rahaman. The assessment of the amount of fat in the human body from measurements of skinfold thickness. *Br. J. Nutr.*, 21:681-689, 1967.

22. Faller, I.L., E.E. Bond, D. Petty, and L.R. Pascale. The use of urinary deuterium oxide and antipyrine dilution methods for measuring total body water in normal and nydropic human subjects. *J. Lab. Clin. Med.*, 45:748-758, 1955.

23. Forbes, G.B. Growth of the lean body mass in man. *Growth*, 36:324-338, 1972.

24. Forbes, G.B. Body composition in adolescence. In *Human Growth* (Vol. 2), edited by F. Falkner and J.M. Tanner. New York: Plenum, 1978.

25. Forbes, G.B., J. Gallup, and J.B. Hursh. Estimation of total body fat from potassium-40 count. *Sci.,* 133:101-102, 1961.

26. Forbes, G.B., and J.B. Hursh. Age and sex trends in lean body mass calculated from K-40 measurements with a note on the theoretical basis for the procedure. *Ann. NY Acad. Sci.,* 110:255-263, 1963.

27. Forbes, G.B., and A.M. Lewis. Total sodium, potassium, and chloride in adult man. *J. Clin. Invest.,* 35:596-600, 1956.

28. Forbes, G.B., F. Schultz, C. Cafarelli, and G.H. Amirhakimi. Effects of body size on potassium-40 measurement in the whole body counter (tilt chair technique). *Health Phys.,* 15:435-442, 1968.

29. Friis-Hansen, B. Body water compartments in children: Changes during growth and related changes in body composition. *Pediat.,* 28:169, 1961.

30. Heald, F.P., E.E. Hunt, R. Schwartz, C.D. Cook, D. Elliot, and B. Vajda. Measures of body fat and hydration in adolescent boys. *Pediat.,* 31:226-239, 1963.

31. Hunt, E.E., and F.P. Heald. Physique of body composition and sexual maturation in adolescent boys. *Ann. NY Acad. Sci.,* 110:532-544, 1963.

32. Johnston, F.E., P.V.V. Hamill, and J. Lemeshow. *Skinfold thickness of youth 12-17 years.* (National Health Survey, Series 11, No. 132, U.S. Dept. of HEW.) Washington: U.S. Government Printing, 1974.

33. Johnston, F.E., P.V.V. Hamill, and J. Lemeshow. *Skinfold thickness of children 6-11 years.* (National Health Survey, Series 11, No. 120, U.S. Dept. of HEW.) Washington: U.S. Government Printing, 1972.

34. Katch, F.I., and W.D. McArdle. Prediction of body density from simple anthropometric measurements in college-age men and women. *Hum. Biol.,* 45:445-453, 1973.

35. Katch, F.E., and E.D. Michael. Densitometric validation of six skinfold formulas to predict body density and percent fat of 17-year-old boys. *Res. Quart.,* 40:712-716, 1969.

36. Keys, A., and J. Brozek. Body fat in adult man. *Physiol. Rev.,* 33:245-325, 1953.

37. Klemm, T., D.H. Banzer, and U. Schneider. Bone mineral content of the growing skeleton. *Amer. J. Roentg.,* 126:1283-1284, 1976.

38. Lesser, G.T., I. Kumar, and J.M. Steele. Changes in body composition with age. *Ann. NY Acad. Sci.,* 110:578-588, 1963.

39. Loeppky, J.A., L.G. Myhre, M.D. Venters, and V.C. Luft. Total body water and lean body mass estimated by ethanol dilution. *J. Appl. Physiol.,* 42:803-808, 1977.

40. Lohman, T.G. Biological variations in body composition. *J. Anim. Sci.,* 32:647-653, 1971.

41. Lohman, T.G., M.H. Slaughter, A. Selinger, and R.A. Boileau. Relationship of body composition to somatotype in college-age men. *Ann. Hum. Biol.,* 5:147-157, 1978.

42. Lohman, T.G. Skinfolds and body density and their relation to body fatness: A review. *Hum. Biol.,* 53:181-225, 1981.

43. Lohman, T.G. Measurements of body composition in children. *J. Phys. Ed. and Rec.,* 53:67-70, 1982.

44. Malina, R.M. Quantification of fat, muscle, and bone in man. *Clin. Orthop.,* 65:9-38, 1969.

45. Malina, R.M. "The measurement of body composition." In *Human physical growth and maturation,* edited by F.E. Johnston, A.F. Roche, and C. Susanne. New York: Plenum, 1980.

46. Matiegka, J. The testing of physical efficiency. *Amer. J. Phys. Anthrop.,* 4:223-230, 1921.

47. Mazess, R.B. Estimation of bone and skeletal weight by direct photon absorptiometry. *Invest. Radiol.,* 6:52-60, 1971.

48. Mazess, R.B., and J.R. Cameron. Skeletal growth in school children's maturation and bone mass. *Amer. J. Phys. Anthrop.,* 35:399-408, 1971.

49. Mazess, R.B., and J.R. Cameron. "Bone mineral content in normal U.S. whites." In *International conference on bone mineral measurement,* edited by R.B. Mazess. (Dept. of HEW Publication No. [NIH] 75-863.) Washington: U.S. Government Printing, 1973.

50. Mazess, R.B., and W. Mather. Bone mineral content of North Alaskan Eskimo. *Amer. J. Clin. Nutr.,* 27:196-226, 1974.

51. Mellits, E.A., and D.B. Cheek. "Growth and body water." In *Human growth: Body composition, cell growth, energy and intelligence,* edited by D.B. Cheek. Philadelphia: Lea & Febiger, 1968.

52. Merz, A.L., M. Trotter, and R.R. Peterson. Estimation of skeletal weight in the living. *Amer. J. Phys. Anthrop.,* 14:589-609, 1956.

53. Moore, F.D., and C.M. Boyden. Body cell mass and limits of hydration of the fat-free body: Their relation to estimated skeletal weight. *Ann. NY Acad. Sci.,* 10:62-71, 1963.

54. Moulton, C.R. Age and chemical development in mammals. *J. Bio. Sci.,* 57:79-97, 1923.

55. Nelp, W.B., H.E. Palmer, R. Meirano, K. Pailthorp, G.M. Hinn, C. Rich, J.L. Williams, T.G. Rudd, and J.D. Denney. Measurement of total body calcium (bone mass) *in vivo* with the use of total body neutron activation and analysis. *J. Lab. Clin. Med.,* 76:151-162, 1970.

56. Novak, L.P. Age and sex differences in body density and creatinine excretion of high school children. *Ann. NY Acad. Sci.,* 110:545-577, 1963.

57. Novak, L.P. Total body water and solids in six- to seven-year-old children: Differences between sexes. *Pediatrics,* 38:483-489, 1966.

58. Osserman, E.F., G.C. Pitts, W.C. Welham, and A.R. Behnke. *In vivo* measurement of body fat and body water in a group of normal men. *J. Appl. Physiol.,* 2:633-639, 1950.

59. Pace, N., L. Kline, H.R. Schachman, and M. Harfenist. Studies of body composition IV. Use of radioactive hydrogen for measurement *in vivo* of total body water. *J. Biol. Chem.,* 168:459-469, 1947.

60. Pace, N., and E. Rathbun. Studies on body composition. *J. Biol. Chem.,* 158:685-691, 1945.

61. Pařizkova, J. Total body fat and skinfold thickness in children. *Metabolism,* 10:794-807, 1961.

62. Pařizkova, J. "Interrelationships between body size, body composition and function." In *Advances in experimental medicine and biology,* edited by A.F. Roche and F. Falkner. New York: Plenum, 1974.

63. Pařizkova, J. Growth and growth velocity of lean body mass and fat in adolescent boys. *Pediatr. Res.,* 10:647-650, 1976.

64. Pascale, L.R., M.I. Grossman, and S. Freeman. *Changes in body composition of soldiers during paratrooper training.* (U.S. Army Medicine Nutrition Laboratory Report No. 150:1-13.) Denver, 1955.

65. Pierson, R.N., D.H.Y. Lin, and R.A. Phillips. Total body potassium in health: Effect of age, sex, height and fat. *Amer. J. Physiol.,* 226:206-212, 1974.

66. Schneider, U., and D. Banzer. "A computerized method of determination of bone mineral content by a transmission scanner." In *International conference on bone mineral measurement,* edited by R.B. Mazess. (Dept. of HEW Publication No. [NIH] 75-863.) Washington: U.S. Government Printing, 1973.

67. Scholerb, P.R., B.J. Friis-Hansen, I.S. Edelman, D.B. Sheldon, and F.D. Moore. The measurement of total body water in the human subject by deuterium oxide dilution. *J. Clin. Invest.,* 37:1296-1310, 1951.

68. Siri, W.E. The gross composition of the body. *Adv. Biol. Med. Phys.,* 4:239-280, 1956.

69. Siri, W.E. "Body composition from fluid spaces and density: Analysis of methods." In *Techniques for measuring body composition,* edited by J. Brozek. Washington: National Academy of Science, 1961.

70. Sloan, A.W. Estimation of body fat in young men. *J. Appl. Physiol.,* 23:311-315, 1967.

71. Sloan, A.W., J.J. Burt, and D.S. Blyth. Estimation of body fat in young women. *J. Appl. Physiol.,* 17:967-970, 1962.

72. Slaughter, M.H., T.G. Lohman, and R.A. Boileau. Relationship of anthropometric dimensions to lean body mass in children. *Ann. Hum. Biol.,* 5:469-482, 1978.

73. Soberman, R., B.B. Brodie, B.B. Levy, J. Axelrod, V. Hollander, and J.M. Steele. The use of antipyrine in the measurement of total body water in man. *J. Biol. Chem.,* 199:31-42, 1949.

74. Spray, C.M., and E.M. Widdowson. The effect of growth and development on the composition of mammals. *Br. J. Nutr.,* 4:332-353, 1950.

75. Trotter, M. A preliminary study of estimation of weight of the skeleton. *Amer. J. Phys. Anthrop.,* 12:537-551, 1954.

76. Trotter, M., G.E. Broman, and R.R. Peterson. Density of cervical vertebrae and comparison with the densities of other bones. *Amer. J. Phys. Anthrop.,* 17:19-25, 1959.

77. Trotter, M., and B.B. Hixon. Sequential changes in weight, density and percentage ash weight of human skeletons from an early fetal period through old age. *Anat. Rec.,* 179:1-18, 1974.

78. West, R.R. The estimation of total skeletal mass from bone densitometry measurements using 60 keV photons. *Br. J. Radiol.,* 46:599-603, 1973.

79. Wilmore, J.H., and A.R. Behnke. Predictability of lean body weight through anthropometric assessment in college men. *J. Appl. Physiol.,* 25:349-355, 1968.

80. Wilmore, J.H., and A.R. Behnke. An anthropometric estimation of body density and lean body weight in young women. *Amer. J. Clin. Nutr.,* 23:267-274, 1970.

81. Womersley, J., K. Boddy, P.C. King, and J.V.G.A. Durnin. A comparison of the fat-free mass of young adults estimated by anthropometry, body density, and total body potassium content. *Clin. Sci.,* 43:469-475, 1972.

82. Womersley, J., J.V.G.A. Durnin, R. Boddy, and M. Mahaffy. Influence of muscular development, obesity and age on the fat-free mass of adults. *J. Appl. Physiol.,* 41:223-229, 1976.

83. Young, C.M., A.D. Bogan, D.A. Roe, and L. Lutwak. Body composition of preadolescent and adolescent girls. IV. Body water and creatinine. *J. Amer. Diet. Assoc.,* 53:579-587, 1968.

3

Human Growth, Maturation, and Regular Physical Activity[1]

Robert M. Malina
University of Texas at Austin

Physical activity is an essential component of the behavioral repertoire of children and youth. Physical activities are the substrate of physical performance, that is, motor skill, muscular strength, and physiological capacities in energy production and work output. They occur in many contexts such as work, leisure, and school, and take many forms in-

[1]This review, with minor revisions, has been published in the June 1983 issue of *Acta Medica Auxologica* and is printed with permission of *Acta Medica Auxologica*.

cluding subsistence (work) activities, exercise as such (calisthenics, running), play and games, dance, and competitive sports. Physical activities thus vary in kind, and their context influences the intensity and duration. In addition, interests in activity and perceived need for physical activity vary with age, sex, biological characteristics, health status, and sociocultural circumstances.

The scope of physical activity and its effect on the human organism is indeed broad. This review will consider only a part of this broad spectrum: the effects of regular physical activity (i.e., training) on selected aspects of physical growth and biological maturation and on specific bodily tissues. This report updates and extends several earlier reviews (55,59,61).

OVERVIEW OF FACTORS
INFLUENCING GROWTH AND MATURATON

The integrated nature of growth and maturation is maintained by the interaction of genes, hormones, nutrients, and the environment in which the individual lives. This complex interaction regulates one's growth and maturation and in general one's physical metamorphosis. An individual's genotype can be viewed as representing potential. Whether a child attains this growth potential, for example, depends on the environment in which he or she is reared. In a growth study, the child is observed in phenotypic form, that is, a product of his/her genotype and environment. The partitioning of genotypic and environmental components in growth and maturation is important to understanding these processes.

Linear body measurements (e.g., stature, leg length) tend to have a higher genetic influence than breadths or circumferences. Circumferences, skinfolds, and body weight have a lower genetic influence than bone dimensions because the former are subject to short-term changes with the environment such as training or nutritional stress. However, the pattern of fat distribution on the body is highly influenced by heredity, as are indices of biological maturity (i.e., menarche, skeletal age, and secondary sex characteristics). Hence, the genetic contribution to individual differences in growth and maturation is significant.

Endocrine secretions are basically regulatory and play an important function in growth and maturation processes. Some growth occurs in the absence of growth-promoting hormones, however, emphasizing the organism's inherent tendency to grow. Endocrine secretions are themselves strongly influenced by genetic mechanisms. These hormones are essential for the full expression of the intrinsic, genetically determined growth and maturation patterns of tissues and systems, and thus the individual. In turn, the nervous system is intimately involved in regulating endocrine secretions, and since the nervous system mediates interactions with the external environments, the sources for potential variation are many.

Interacting with the child's genotype and endocrine secretions is his/her nutritional status. Nutrient requirements are many and, from the developmental perspective, they can be viewed in terms of energy and proteins for growth, maintenance, and repair. Nutrient requirements vary considerably with age, sex, and body size, and in the growing organism they vary with stage of growth. The energy needs to support growth are greatest during infancy and progressively decline with age. On the other hand, the energy needs for maintenance increase during growth. In other words, as the individual gets bigger, more energy is needed to support this size. However, the rate of growth declines with age so that the amount of energy required to support the growth processes per se is progressively reduced.

Having briefly reviewed the major factors influencing a child's growth and maturation, let us consider other factors that influence growth — factors whose direct effects are more difficult to identify or which are of less overall importance. Of these, the role of physical activity is often viewed as a favorable influence on the growth and maturation of children. It should be noted, however, that physical activity is only one of many factors that may affect growth and maturation; so the precise role of properly graded activity programs in influencing these processes is not completely understood.

Physical Activity and Training

Physical activity is not necessarily the same as regular physical training. Although they are obviously a part of training programs, not all physical activities quality as training. Physical training refers to the regular, systematic practice of specific physical activities such as calisthenics, lifting weights, isometric exercises, running, and games/sports activities performed at specific intensities and for specific durations. Training programs vary in kind or type: endurance training, strength training, sprint training, and skill training. The effects of such programs are generally specific to the type of training stimulus (10,21,28,66,82,85), although training effects induced by one kind of program may be more general. For example, running apparently has more general effects than cycling. Training is not a single entity, then, but varies in kind, intensity, and duration. It can be viewed as a continuum, ranging from relatively mild work to severely stressing activity.

In studies of training during growth, programs vary in type, intensity, and duration and are often described simply as mild, moderate, or severe. Youngsters sometimes are simply defined as "active" or "inactive." These labels may be based upon teacher and/or coach assessment, frequency and duration of sport participation, and self-reported activity levels. There is thus a need to qualify and quantify training programs such as number of sessions per week, duration of workouts, number of meters swum during a workout and at what intensity, and number of miles run per workout and at what time or pace. Age-group swimmers (ages 9-12) in some programs may swim about 4,500 meters per session at varying time intervals 6 days per week, while in other programs they may swim only 2,500 meters per session.

Study Designs

Data from a variety of studies have been used to make inferences about the effects of regular physical activity on human growth and maturation.

1. Experimental studies compare trained (treatment) and untrained (control) groups. Because the training stimulus usually varies in type, intensity, and duration, it is difficult to define and quantify the training stimulus within and across studies. Selection of subjects, motivation to train, and control of outside activity are also critical factors. In addition, variable and composite age groups of children and youth are used and the samples tend to be small. Attrition rates tend to be high, and most studies are only short-term. Lacking are experimental studies in which the training factor has been regularly applied and the changes monitored over a sufficient time period during growth. Difficulties inherent in conducting longitudinal programs with children and youth are obvious. Hence, a significant amount of experimental data are derived by extrapolation from studies of animals. Although reasonable generalizations can be made for human growth, the concept of species specificity must be recognized.

A drawback of studies that monitor changes associated with regular training during youth is that they do not ordinarily focus on the growth and maturation of children. Instead, many studies focus on physiological changes associated with training such as maximal oxygen consumption and metabolic substrates. Growth observations are usually made indirectly or in passing, while maturity status is generally not even considered.

2. Comparisons of athletes and nonathletes during childhood and adolescence are commonly used to make inferences about the effects of physical training on growth and maturation. It is assumed that the athletes had been training regularly, and differences in growth and maturation relative to nonathletes are attributed to the training programs required for the specific sports. Problems with such an approach are subject selection and the definition of an athlete at a young age. Youngsters proficient in sports are undoubtedly selected for skill and, in some sports, for size. Size, physique, strength, and motor skill proficiency are related (56,65), and an individual's strength and motor ability may in turn influence his/her level of habitual activity. Maturity differences also

characterize youngsters who excel in sports, and these differences are especially apparent during puberty (62,63). Males who are successful in sports competition are usually somewhat advanced biologically. This probably reflects the size, strength, and performance advantages associated with earlier biological maturation (56). In contrast, females who excel in sports tend to be average or late in biological maturity status with swimmers tending toward the average while female athletes in other sports tend to be late maturing (62,63). Late maturing girls tend to be leaner and more linear in physique, factors that may be more suitable for sports performance.

Nevertheless, young athletes of both sexes grow as well as nonathletes do; the experience of athletic training and competition has neither harmful nor stimulatory effects on statural growth and biological maturation. Regular training does influence the body weight and composition of young athletes. This is discussed later in the chapter. However, maturity-associated variation in size and body composition is a significant factor in comparing athletes and nonathletes, especially during puberty.

Another factor which must be considered in comparing young athletes and nonathletes is the role of social circumstances, that is, socialization into or away from sports. Social factors may interact or vary with a youngster's growth and maturity progress and in turn influence his/her choice of sports or activities (63).

3. Comparisons of adult athletes with nonathletes or the general population are also used to make inferences on the effects of regular physical activity during growth. It is assumed that the adult athletes began training during their youth, and that the differences relative to nonathletes reflect training effects on growth and maturation processes. Most recently, such an approach was used to make inferences on the effects of early training on the sexual maturation of young girls (30). Problems associated with subject selection, age of onset of training, and motivation to persist in training programs are similar to those already mentioned.

4. Some activities require extreme levels of unilateral effort, such as tennis, baseball pitching, and specific manual occupations. Such specialized activity is occasionally used to illustrate training effects. The individual is his/her own control, as the dominant limb (trained) is compared to the nondominant limb (untrained). Observations from such studies are ordinarily limited to the skeletal and muscular aspects of the upper extremity.

5. The co-twin control method involves comparisons of identical twins who are discordant for regular physical activity. One twin is regularly trained while the other is not, but instead follows his/her usual pattern of activity. Data from such studies primarily consider physiological variables (37,38,98).

6. Clinical and experimental observations of prolonged bed rest, im-

mobilization with casts, and muscular inactivation as in nerve injuries also lend insights into the role of physical activity in developing and maintaining the integrity of skeletal and muscular tissues. These are perhaps most apparent in the muscular atrophy and loss of skeletal mineral associated with prolonged inactivity or disuse.

Developmental Trends in Activity Habits

Studies on the effects of training during childhood and youth are confounded in part by problems associated with any attempt to partition training-induced effects from those changes which accompany normal growth and maturation. It is essential to monitor the effects of regular activity over and above normal childhood activity. Measures or estimates of "normal" activity are limited in scope and are primarily based upon surveys of sport activities of adolescents with little data for pre-adolescents.

Renson and colleagues (77), for example, considered the sporting activity of a large, mixed longitudinal sample of Belgian boys ages 12 through 18. Boys were placed into one of four categories based upon the hours of active sport involvement per week over a 1-year period. The percentage of boys in the inactive category (0-1 hr/week) decreased from ages 12 through 18, while the percentage in the very active category (> 6 hr/week) increased. The percentage of boys in the moderately active group (1-3 hr/week) showed only a slight decrease, while the percentage in the active group (3-6 hr/week) showed a moderate increase from 12 to 18 years of age. In a longitudinal study of West German adolescents (25 girls and 26 boys), Ilmarinen and Rutenfranz (41) used four annual retrospective interviews with a standardized questionnaire. There was a definite decrease in yearly sport activity in both sexes from ages 14 to 17. Boys decreased sporting activity by 70% between 15 and 17 years of age, whereas the corresponding value for girls was 57%, most of the decrease occurring from 14 to 15 years of age. Comparison of the sport activity scores between the sexes indicated a total sport activity score for boys that was about four times greater than that for girls at 15 years of age, but only two times greater at 17 years of age. Similar age and sex differences were apparent when sport activity scores were viewed on a monthly basis.

Engström (23) considered the attitude toward and the scope of physical activity (hours per week) in a sample of Swedish males and females at 15, 20, and 25 years of age (22% drop-out in the original sample). The youth and young adults expressed very positive attitudes toward physical activity, but the amount of activity did not correspond to this attitude. The average hours of physical activity per week for boys decreased from 4.8 hours at 15 years to 2.6 hours at 20 years, and then increased to about 2.9 hours per week at 25 years of age. Corresponding values for girls were 3.3 hours per week at 15 years, 1.8 hours per week at 20 years, and 2.2 hours per week at 25 years of age. The decrease from 15 to 20 years of age in both sexes (46%) may relate to adolescence itself, with its concomitant social demands and career decisions.

Activity and Stature

Regular physical activity has no apparent effect on stature in growing individuals. Although some early data suggest that an increase in stature occurs with regular training (1,6,86), the observed changes are usually quite small and are derived from studies that did not control for subject selection and for maturity status at the time of training or at the time of making the comparisons. The study by Åstrand et al. (4) on the growth and functional capacity of elite female swimmers is often cited as suggesting that training stimulates growth in stature. A close examination of the data for the 30 swimmers, however, indicates that the girls in fact had been taller than the average since 7 years of age and apparently entered adolescence slightly earlier than the Swedish reference data for the 1950s. Mean stature was +0.4 standard deviation units at 7 years of age and +0.6 standard deviation units at the time of the study when the girls ranged in age from 11.9 to 16.4 years. The apparent acceleration in statural growth was not related to the intensity of training. Rather, it was probably related to the swimmers' somewhat earlier maturation. eight girls attained menarche between 11.0 and 11.9 years of age, seven between 12.0 and 12.9, 10 between 13.0 and 13.9, and four after 14.0 years. The average age at menarche for the group was 12.9 years; therefore, since menarche generally follows peak height velocity, one might expect the young swimmers to be somewhat taller. Their tallness probably represents earlier maturation and not the effects of intensive swimming training. Our studies of elite young female swimmers (64,68) also indicate that they are taller than the reference data and approximate the reference data in the timing of menarche.

In a study of young boys (11-13 years of age) selected for swimming training, Milicer and Denisiuk (69) noted slightly greater average increments in stature over 2 years of training compared to a control sample. The apparent rate differences in statural growth most likely reflect maturity variation. The young swimmers included a greater percentage of early maturers (25%) compared to the control sample (17%), and did not include any late maturers. Our observations on male age-group swimmers from 8 to 17 years of age (67) indicate mean statures larger than the reference data and somewhat advanced development of secondary sex characteristics.

Three studies that assessed the effects of endurance running training on boys between 10 and 15 years of age (20,22,24) did not include measures of maturity status, although the boys' statures at the start of training corresponded to accepted reference data. In Ekblom's (22) study, five boys (age 11 at the start) trained for 32 months and showed a somewhat accelerated growth rate in stature compared to Swedish reference data. In contrast, the control group of four boys did not. It is difficult to consider the accelerated growth relative to training, as maturity status was not controlled and the boys could have experienced all or part of their adolescent spurts, given the normal variation in timing and intensity of the male adolescent growth spurt (90).

Eriksson's (24) observations were similar. The 12 boys in the sample, 11 to 13 years of age, increased on the average 3.5 cm in stature after 16 weeks of endurance training. However, an average gain of 3.5 cm over 4 months would correspond to an annual gain of about 10 cm, which would seem to suggest the adolescent growth spurt. Since maturity status was not controlled, it is difficult to ascertain whether the observed changes are the result of training or simply reflect normal adolescent growth. The six boys (10-15 years of age) followed by Daniels and Oldridge (20) trained for 22 months in endurance running. Their statures equaled the reference data at the start of the study but, in contrast to the above studies, were slightly below the standard at the termination.

Although the preceding review indicates that regular training does not stimulate growth in stature, it is also apparent that the experience of training and competition in sports does not have a negative effect on statural growth. This is relevant to the frequently misquoted early study by Rowe (80), who compared the growth in stature and weight of male athletes and nonathletes, 13.7 to 15.7 years of age, over a 2-year period. Rowe noted that the athletes were taller but grew at a slower rate over the 2-year period. Some have taken this observation at face value (54,76,87) without heeding Rowe's (80) qualifying comment that the observed differences could reflect differential timing of the adolescent spurt: "Since the athletic group is composed of boys who have matured earlier, age considered, than the group of non-athletic boys, the athletic boy is not going to grow as much as the non-athletic boy over the period studied" (p. 115).

It is apparent that the literature is based almost entirely on generally small samples of the growth of youngsters participating in sport activities. Similar results were revealed (78,81) in comparisons of larger samples of youth, including both athletes and nonathletes grouped by degree of physical activity.

Activity, Body Weight, and Body Composition

Regular physical activity is an important factor in the regulation and maintenance of body weight. Body weight is a heterogenous mass, quite often partitioned into lean body mass and fat. Regular training generally results in an increase in lean body mass and a corresponding decrease in body fat in children and youth. Training produces similar effects in adults, quite often without any appreciable change in body weight (74). However, results are not consistent across studies (26). The magnitude of change in body composition with regular activity varies with the intensity and duration of the program, and the changes are dependent on continued activity. For example, Pařizkova (74) reported fluctuations in body fatness and density which were proportional to the intensity of training in young gymnasts (n = 10, ages 13-18) followed longitudinally over 5 years. Fat levels decreased as the girls engaged in training for the competitive season, and increased once again as training tapered.

Body composition changes considerably during normal growth and maturation so that it becomes difficult to separate effects of training from those associated with normal growth. Further, the continuity of fatness levels from childhood through adolescence is rather weak (18), which emphasizes the variation in fatness associated with growth and maturation.

In one of the more comprehensive studies of training and body composition, Pařizkova (74) followed boys engaged in different levels of sports participation and training over the 7-year period from 11 to 18 years of age. Three levels of training were compared: regularly trained (intensive, 6 hr/week); trained but not on a regular basis (in sport schools, about 4 hours of organized exercise per week), and untrained (about 2.5 hr/week, including school physical education). Sample sizes for the three groups at the end of the study were small, however, 8, 18, and 13, respectively. The groups did not differ in anthropometric characteristics nor in body composition at the beginning of the study. During and after the study the most active boys had significantly more lean body mass and less fat than the least and moderately active boys, who differed only slightly among themselves.

Von Dobëln and Eriksson (95) reported significant body composition changes in nine boys (ages 11-13) after an endurance training program. Using potassium measurements, they observed average gains of 0.5 kg in weight and 12 grams in potassium at the end of the training program. A 12-gram increase in potassium corresponds to a gain of about 4 kg of muscle mass, which would indicate that the 0.5 kg gain in body weight was accompanied by a loss of about 3 kg of fat during the training program. Relative to statural growth, the increase in potassium was about 6% greater than expected while the gain in body weight was about 5% less than expected. These changes are perhaps the result of training and growth since the boys gained, on the average, 3.5 cm in stature over the 16-week program (24, see section on stature), which may indicate that the adolescent spurt occurred during the program. Also, male adolescence is accompanied by a significant increase in muscle mass.

The results of these two studies summarize quite well the information on training and body composition. Youngsters who regularly engage in

physical activity programs, either formal training for sport or recreational activities, are generally leaner; they have more lean body mass and less
fat than those who are not regularly active (64,78,81). Two questions remain, however: Are the changes in body composition associated with
regular activity greater than those associated with normal growth and
maturation? How persistent are the training-associated changes? The increase in lean body mass observed in youths who train regularly for
several years would seem to suggest an increase greater than expected
with normal growth. However, it should be noted that muscle mass, and
thus lean body mass, continues to increase into the mid-20s. On the other
hand, most of the variation in body composition with activity or inactivity is associated with fatness, which fluctuates inversely with the training
stimulus. Changes in response to short-term training programs are most
likely related to fluctuating levels of fatness, with only minimal changes
in lean body mass.

Methods of estimating body composition *in vivo* are indirect, and
most are based upon models derived from adults (60). Hence, it must be
recognized that the estimates reported in any study include a certain
degree of measurement variability. Such error is especially significant in
longitudinal studies where it may be compounded in repeated measurement sessions. In addition, prediction equations are sometimes used to
monitor body composition changes with training. However, evidence indicates that equations based upon skinfolds may not be sufficiently sensitive to detect lean body mass changes with training (99).

Activity and Physique

Physique refers to the general configuration of the whole body as opposed to emphasis on specific features. The concept of somatotype is
used most often in developmental studies. It is a composite based on
varying contributions of three components: endomorphy (fatness),
mesomorphy (skeletal and muscular development), and ectomorphy
(linearity). Pařizkova and Carter (75) considered the stability of anthropometric estimates of somatotypes in the sample of 39 boys followed
longitudinally from ages 11 to 18 by Pařizkova (74, see body composition section). The three groups of boys experienced different levels of
regular physical activity during this period. The distribution of
somatotypes did not differ among the three activity groups, suggesting
no effect of the training programs on somatotype. Rather, individuals
changed considerably in somatotype over the 7-year period. Changes occurred in a random manner and were not attributable to physical activity. All boys changed in somatotype ratings at least once, and 67%
changed in component dominance. Thus, individual variation in
somatotype stability during adolescence confounds the evaluation of
possible training-related changes. In a follow-up of a subsample (n = 14)

of the original series at 24 years of age, mesomorphy had increased between the ages of 18 to 24 even though the boys had ceased regular training (13).

Several studies of teenagers (55,61) indicate beneficial effects of short-term training on muscular development, especially in those body parts specifically trained such as thoracic and arm measurements of gymnasts, muscular development in the shoulder region of swimmers, and muscular development in response to weight training.

Activity and Skeletal Maturation

Although regular activity functions to enhance skeletal mineralization and density (see below), it does not accelerate or delay skeletal maturity as assessed in growth studies, that is, initial ossification, shape changes in epiphyseal centers, and eventual union of epiphyses and diaphyses in the hand-wrist. Černy (14) monitored the skeletal maturity of the boys engaged in the training project of Pařizkova (74) discussed earlier. There were no skeletal maturity differences among the three groups before, during, and after the study. Rather, variation in skeletal maturity within the different activity groups was greater than between. Kotulán and colleagues (50) considered skeletal maturity in a sample of young male athletes followed longitudinally from 12 to 15 years of age. The boys trained regularly for cycling, rowing, and ice hockey. Over the 3-year period, the gains in skeletal maturity varied between 2.6 and 3.3 years in the athletes; these gains in skeletal maturity did not differ from control subjects (3.2 years) and young athletes who started the training program but dropped out (3.3 years).

In a sample of elite female athletes including gymnasts, figure skaters, tennis players, volleyball players, and football players, Novotny (71) assessed their skeletal maturity initially and after 3 or 4 years of regular training. The young athletes were rated as advanced, normal, or retarded in skeletal maturity. After the period of regular training, only 19 (21%) of the 89 girls changed categories, while 70 (79%) remained in the same skeletal maturity category. Of the small number who changed categories, 11 shifted from advanced to normal or from normal to delayed, while 8 shifted from delayed to normal or from normal to advanced. In addition, at the beginning and end of the study, mean chronological and skeletal ages of the young athletes did not differ significantly. The results of these three studies from Czechoslovakia would thus seem to indicate that skeletal maturity as assessed in growth studies is not affected by regular physical training in young adolescent boys and girls.

Activity and Sexual Maturation

Intensive physical training has been suggested as a factor which may delay menarche, that is, sexual maturation of young girls (see 63 for a comprehensive review). The data dealing with intensive training and menarche are quite limited, associational, speculative, and do not control for other factors which influence the time of menarche. Inferences on the role of training are largely based upon the observation that menarche occurs, on the average, later in athletes in general than in nonathletes, and later in those who began training prior to the maturational event than in those who began training after menarche.

The relationship between training and menarche is currently of considerable interest, given the conclusion of Frisch et al. (30:1582) "that intense physical activity does in fact delay menarche." This conclusion is based upon a small sample of university athletes, 12 swimmers and 6 runners, who began training before menarche. The correlation between age at menarche and years of training before menarche was +0.53, a moderate relationship. However, note that correlation indicates only a relationship between the two variables and does not imply a cause-effect sequence. It could have been that the young women undertook training because of their delayed maturation rather than the training delaying their maturation. Our data for a small sample of Olympic volleyball players ($n = 18$) shows no correlation ($r = -0.05$) between age at menarche and duration of training before menarche (63).

The suggested mechanism for the association between intensive training and menarche is hormonal. It is suggested that training influences levels of gonadotrophic and ovarian hormones, which in turn delays menarche. The endocrine data offered to support this notion, however, are derived largely from studies of women, both athletes and nonathletes, case studies, and extremely small samples, who have already attained menarche. The evidence indicates short-term increments in hormonal levels, including almost all gonadotrophic and sex steroid hormones, with training. What is specifically relevant for premenarcheal girls is the possible cumulative effects of hormonal responses to regular training. Such data are presently lacking.

A corollary of the suggestion that training delays menarche is that the weight or body composition changes associated with training may function to delay menarche, that is, delay maturity of young girls by keeping them lean. This, in turn, is related to the critical weight or fatness hypothesis (29) that a certain level of fatness is needed for menarche to occur. This hypothesis has been discussed at length by many researchers (42,57,93), the conclusion being that the data do not support the specificity of weight or fatness as the critical variable for menarche.

There is a moderately high correlation between age at menarche and skeletal maturity, and a reduced variance in skeletal ages at the time of menarche (57,90). Further, the process of skeletal maturation is influenced by gonadal hormones, among others. Thus, if the hormonal responses to regular training influence sexual maturation, one might expect them to also influence skeletal maturation during puberty. This is clearly not the case in the three studies of training and skeletal maturity already discussed.

Activity and Specific Tissues

The focus of the preceding discussion is the effects of regular physical activity on biological growth and maturation. These are biological processes, but we ordinarily do not study the processes per se. Rather, observations are based on the outcomes of the underlying developmental processes. For example, stature is a composite measurement involving many growth loci, but we do not measure the processes at the growth plates of specific long bones or vertebrae. In a similar manner, we observe stages of skeletal maturation and not the process of ossification occurring in a specific bone. Or in the case of menarche, emphasis is on the presence or absence of this developmental event, not on the processes leading to the beginning of the menses.

There is reasonably extensive literature in the exercise and sport sciences that considers the effects of activity programs on specific tissues and functions. Many of these efforts are approaching the level at which developmental processes occur, and may thus contribute to our understanding of regular activity on the processes of growth and maturation. The subsequent discussion considers some of the information dealing with the effects of regular training on bone, muscle, and fat tissues.

Bone. Experimental studies of developing animals (45,47,83,84) indicate greater skeletal mineralization and density, and wider, more robust bones with prolonged physical training. Observations on adult humans engaged in prolonged unilateral activity as in tennis (12,40,43) or baseball pitching (46,94) indicate similar results, that is, wider, more robust bones, and increased bone mineral in the preferred arm compared to the nonpreferred arm. Since the majority of adults began formal training during childhood, the evidence would suggest a training-mediated response. Activity-related bone mineralization data for children are limited. In a study of bone mineralization of the dominant and nondominant arms of amateur baseball players 8 to 19 years of age, Watson (97) reported significant mineralization and width differences between the dominant and nondominant humeri, but not for the radii and ulnae. The differences in mineral content between the dominant and nondominant humeri increased with age, which would suggest a training effect, assuming that the older boys participated in the specialized throwing activity longer than the younger boys in the sample.

It should be noted that these studies of unilateral activities indicate rather localized increases in bone mineralization. In a comparison of the densities of the distal femora of young adult athletes and nonathletes, Nilsson and Westlin (70) noted greater femoral densities in the athletes and a clear gradient of highest densities in the "top" athletes through the "ordinary" athletes, and exercising controls to the nonexercising subjects. Dalen and Olsson (19) observed a 20% increase in the trabecular bone of the extremities among cross-country runners, while Aloia et al. (2) found an increased total bone mass in marathon runners. It is suggested that the differences relative to nonrunners may represent beneficial effects of regular physical activity on bone mineralization during growth.

Experimental literature on training and specific bone lengths indicates reduced bone lengths in rats (52,92) and mice (45) exposed to voluntary or forced swimming and moderate or intensive running. Corresponding data for humans are not available. The observations of Kato and Ishiko (44) suggest that excessive compressive forces on the epiphyses of the knee may obstruct growth and thus reduce stature. The sample upon which this suggestion is based, however, came from an economically poor and nutritionally substandard background. The experimental and clinical data of Viteri and Torun (96), on the other hand, suggest that regular activity during rehabilitation from protein-energy malnutrition facilitates recovery, including linear growth. Buskirk et al. (12) reported longer bones of the dominant arm compared to the nondominant arm of elite tennis players, and suggested that the difference is attributable to the effects of vigorous activity on bone growth during the adolescent years.

Given the evidence on activity and growth of a bone in length, it seems that the conclusion of Steinhaus (89), presented about 50 years ago, may still be plausible: The pressure effects of physical activity may stimulate epiphyseal growth to an optimal length, but excessive pressure can retard linear growth. There is obvious need to evaluate the effects of activity on the epiphyseal growth plate. When dealing with youngsters, it is difficult to define excessive pressure. As noted earlier, elite young athletes apparently grow as well in stature as do nonathletes even after controlling for maturity differences and recognizing the possible role of selection for small body size in some sports.

Muscle. Growth of muscle tissue postnatally is characterized by constancy in number of muscle fibers, an increase in fiber size, and a considerable increase in number of muscle nuclei which are apparently derived from satellite cells (58). Regular physical training commonly results in hypertrophy of skeletal muscle. The degree of hypertrophy varies with the intensity of the training stimulus and it appears that "increased tension development (either passive or active) is the critical event in initiating compensatory growth" of skeletal muscle (31:248). Hypertrophy is accompanied by an increase in contractile substances (35), myofibrils (32), enzyme activity (36), and strength. The concept of the specificity of training must be emphasized, as muscular hypertrophy is associated primarily with high-resistance training activities such as weight training and may not occur with endurance training. Hypertrophy occurs in the existing muscle fibers and not as a result of an increase in the number of fibers. However, some experimental evidence with adult animals indicates that muscle fibers will divide by longitudinal fission (fiber splitting) under the stress of excessive, prolonged training (34), although other data are not consistent with these observations. Other evidence for adult experimental animals also indicates training-induced increases in DNA levels and presumably the number of muscle nuclei in skeletal muscle (15).

The specificity of training is well documented and several examples will suffice. After 5 months of endurance training in six adult males, Gollnick et al. (33) noted no change in the percentages of slow- and fast-twitch fibers, and an increase in succinate dehydrogenase (SDH) and phosphofructokinase (PFK) activities by 95% and 11%, respectively. SDH activity is an indicator of the oxidative potential of the fibers, while PFK is regarded as the rate-limiting enzyme for glycolysis. SDH activity (oxidative potential) increased in both the fast- and slow-twitch fibers, while PFK activity (glycolytic capacity) apparently increased only in fast-twitch fibers. In contrast, the relative area of the muscle composed of slow-twitch fibers increased with endurance training.

Using an 8-week front crawl swimming program as the training stimulus, Lavoie et al. (53) observed no changes in fiber distribution and in SDH and PFK activities in seven young adult males (recreational swimmers, not formally trained in competitive swimming). However, the relative area of fast-twitch fibers increased significantly as did the ratio of fast- to slow-twitch fibers. With an 8-week progressive strength training program in 14 adult males, Thorstensson (91) observed no change in the percentage distribution of fast-twitch and slow-twitch fibers. However, changes in the ratio of fast- to slow-twitch fiber area suggested a specific hypertrophy of fast-twitch fibers with strength training. On the other hand, the strength training program had an insignificant effect on selected "contractility" enzymes, that is myokinase and creatine phosphokinase. Krotkiewski et al. (51) reported generally similar results after 5 weeks of strength training in 10 adult women. There were increases in muscle thickness (especially in the area of fast-twitch fibers), and in myokinase and lactate dehydrogenase activities in the exercised leg compared to the nonexercised leg.

Data on muscle tissue responses to training in developing organisms is not as extensive as that for adults. Nevertheless, results of several studies are in a similar direction as those for adults. There is a need to more carefully consider the effects of different kinds of training on the muscle tissue in developing organisms so that training-associated changes can perhaps be distinguished from those that accompany normal growth.

Studies of high-resistance weight training in children and youth indicate muscular hypertrophy of the exercised muscle groups (55). Persistence of the changes after training ceases is not ordinarily considered. Studies of DNA content, and thus number of muscle nuclei in growing animals undergoing regular training, indicate a significant rise in DNA above that expected from normal growth (5,11,39). The normal pattern of change in DNA content of skeletal muscle tissue with growth is one of a steady increase until puberty with a rather constant level thereafter. The increased DNA in trained animals would seem to suggest that training is a significant factor influencing nuclear number during growth.

Among five boys 11 years of age who were endurance trained for 6 weeks, Eriksson (24,25) observed no change in the muscle fiber population of the muscle tissue sampled but did note a marked increase in the oxidative potential of both slow- and fast-twitch fibers. SDH activity increased 30%, while PFK activity increased 83%, a marked increase with the short-term training program. It should be noted that PFK activity in the boys was low compared to adult values, which would suggest differences in magnitude of response between developing individuals and adults. More recently, Fournier et al. (27) compared the responses of 12 adolescent boys, 16 to 17 years of age, to 3 months of sprint and endurance training and 6 months of detraining. There were no changes in fiber distribution in both groups, but the endurance trained group showed an increase in the surface area of slow- and fast-twitch fibers. The sprint trained group demonstrated no change in fiber surface area. A 42% increase in SDH activity and no change in PFK activity was observed in the endurance trained group. In contrast, the sprint trained group had a 21% increase in PFK activity and no change in SDH activity.

After 6 months of detraining, SDH activity in the endurance trained group and PFK activity in the sprint trained group fell to lower values than at the start of training; however, the mean values did not differ significantly. The results of both studies thus illustrate the specificity of training in youth and demonstrate responses which are similar in direction to those observed in adults. However, the magnitude of the responses differ.

Results of the studies on youth and adults indicate that the distribution of fiber types is not altered by training. This would suggest that genetic factors are of primary significance in determining skeletal muscle fiber distribution, and the data for twins would support this conclusion (9). However, the relative area of a muscle composed of slow- or fast-twitch fibers may change in response to training with the direction of change depending on the type of training stimulus. Thus, although genetic factors are important in determining the fiber composition of muscle tissue, the evidence emphasizes the importance of physical training in modifying the metabolic capacity.

Adipose. Given the current interest in adipose tissue cellularity during growth (16,17,49,79), and the generally favorable influence of training on body fatness (see above), one can inquire into the possible effects of regular training during growth on adipose tissue cellularity. Björntorp et al. (7), for example, reported a training-associated reduction in fat cell size in young adult soccer players and middle-age endurance athletes. Krotkiewski et al. (51), on the other hand, observed a reduction in subcutaneous fat thickness with strength training in adult women, but no significant changes in estimated fat cell size. Rather, the evidence suggested that the decreased thickness of subcutaneous tissue was a function of altered muscle thickness, i.e., "the same fat now surrounds an increased muscle volume" (51:279).

Some experimental evidence suggests that training initiated early in the life of rats (at preweaning ages) effectively reduced the rate of fat cell accumulation and thus resulted in a significant reduction in the number of fat cells and body fatness later in life (72,73). On the other hand, endurance running begun after 7 weeks of age in rats did not affect adipose cell number, but it significantly reduced adipose cell size (3,8). These results thus indicate an important role for regular activity in regulating fat cell size; however, in order for training to influence fat cell number the program must be initiated very early in the life of rats. By about 7 weeks of age, the pattern of fat cell proliferation in rats is apparently established so that adipose cells continue to increase in number even though a training stimulus may be present.

It is not certain whether the preceding experimental observations can be applied to developing children. If so, training programs may need to be initiated early in life to have an influence on adipose tissue cellularity. However, the present information on developmental age trends and sex differences and regional variability in estimated adipose cell number and size is variable across studies (48,59).

CONCLUDING REMARKS

Only selected aspects of physical growth and maturation relative to the stress of regular physical training have been considered. Other areas of research are undoubtedly relevant. Changes in aerobic power during growth and under the influence of training have been reviewed recently by Bouchard et al. (10) and are further considered in this volume. There is a need for more detailed examination of hormonal responses to regular training and their possible relationships to growth and maturation. Growth hormone responses to physical activity have been reviewed by Shephard and Sidney (88) and Malina (59). A closer examination of gonadotrophic and gonadal hormone responses to regular training is needed especially since such responses are implicated in a possible relationship between training and sexual maturation (63).

Regular physical training has no apparent effect on stature in growing individuals and on biological maturation as commonly assessed in growth studies. On the other hand, regular physical activity is a significant factor in the regulation of body weight and composition, and in the growth and integrity of skeletal and muscle tissues. The role of regular activity in the development of adipose tissue cellularity is not clearly established, although activity will function to reduce fatness. More active individuals generally show greater changes in fat and lean tissues with training, but some training-associated changes are specific to the type of program followed.

Physical activity is apparently essential for normal growth; it is not known just how much activity is necessary during the years of active growth. The role of regular activity in the biological maturation process is not clearly established. There is a need to develop sensitive methods of monitoring and quantifying the amount and intensity of normal physical activity in children and youth. Further studies that employ different training programs are obviously necessary, especially longitudinal observations of childen and youth for whom the training stimulus is carefully defined and quantified.

REFERENCES

1. Adams, E.H. A comparative anthropometric study of hard labor during youth as a stimulator of physical growth of young colored women. *Res. Quart.,* 9:102-108, 1938.

2. Aloia, J.F., S.H. Cohn, T. Babu, C. Abesamis, N. Kalici, and K. Ellis. Skeletal mass and body composition in marathon runners. *Metabolism,* 27:1793-1796, 1978.

3. Askew, E.W., and A.L. Hecker. Adipose tissue cell size and lipolysis in the rat: Response to exercise intensity and food restriction. *J. Nutr.,* 106:1351-1360, 1976.

4. Åstrand, P.-O., L. Engström, B.O. Eriksson, P. Carlberg, I. Nylander, B. Saltin, and C. Thoren. Girl swimmers. *Acta Paediatr. Scand. Suppl.,* 147:1-75, 1963.

5. Bailey, D.A., R.D. Bell, and R.E. Howarth. The effect of exercise on DNA and protein synthesis in skeletal muscle of growing rats. *Growth,* 37:323-331, 1973.

6. Beyer, H.G. The influence of exercise on growth. *J. Exp. Med.,* 1:546-558, 1896.

7. Björntorp, P., G. Grimby, H. Sanne, L. Sjostrøm, G. Tibblin, and L. Wilhelmsen. Adipose tissue fat cell size in relation to metabolism in

weight-stabile, physically active men. *Hormone Met. Res.,* 4:178-182, 1972.

8. Booth, M.A., M.J. Booth, and A.W. Taylor. Rat fat cell size and number with exercise training, detraining and weight loss. *Fed. Proc.,* 33:1959-1963, 1974.

9. Bouchard, C., and R.M. Malina. "Genetics of physiological fitness and motor performance." In *Exercise and sport science reviews* (Vol. eleven), edited by R.L. Terjung, pp. 306-339. Philadelphia: Franklin Institute Press, 1983.

10. Bouchard, C., M.-C. Thibault, and J. Jobin. Advances in selected areas of human work physiology. *Yrbk. Phys. Anthropol.,* 24:1-36, 1981.

11. Buchanan, T.A.S., and J.J. Pritchard. DNA content of tibialis anterior of male and female white rats measured from birth to 50 weeks. *J. Anat.,* 107:185, 1970.

12. Buskirk, E.R., K.L. Andersen, and J. Brožek. Unilateral activity and bone and muscle development in the forearm. *Res. Quart.,* 27:127-131, 1956.

13. Carter, J.E.L., and J. Pařizkova. Changes in somatotypes of European males between 17 and 24 years. *Amer. J. Phys. Anthropol.,* 48:251-254, 1978.

14. Cěrny, L. "The results of an evaluation of skeletal age of boys 11-15 years old with different regime of physical activity." In *Physical fitness assessment,* edited by V. Seliger, pp. 56-59. Prague: Charles University, 1969.

15. Christensen, D.A., and E.W. Crampton. Effects of exercise and diet on nitrogenous constituents in several tissues of adult rats. *J. Nutr.,* 86:369-375, 1965.

16. Chumlea, W.C., J.L. Knittle, A.F. Roche, R.M. Siervogel, and P. Webb. Size and number of adipocytes and measures of body fat in boys and girls 10 to 18 years of age. *Amer. J. Clin. Nutr.,* 34:1791-1797, 1981.

17. Chumlea, W.C., R.M. Siervogel, A.F. Roche, D. Mukherjee, and P. Webb. Changes in adipocyte cellularity in children ten to 18 years of age. *Int. J. Obesity,* 6:383-389, 1982.

18. Cronk, C.E., A.F. Roche, R. Kent, D. Eichorn, and R.W. McCammon. Longitudinal trends in subcutaneous fat thickness during adolescence. *Amer. J. Phys. Anthropol.,* 61:197-204, 1983.

19. Dalen, N., and K.E. Olsson. Bone mineral content and physical activity. *Acta Orthop. Scand.,* 45:170-174, 1974.

20. Daniels, J., and N. Oldridge. Changes in oxygen consumption of young boys during growth and running training. *Med. Sci. Sports,* 3:161-165, 1971.

21. Edgerton, V.R. Neuromuscular adaptation to power and endurance work. *Can. J. Appl. Sport Sci.,* 1:49-58, 1976.

22. Ekblom, B. Effect of physical training on oxygen transport system in man. *Acta Physiol. Scand. Suppl.*, 328:1-45, 1969.

23. Engström, L.M. Physical activity of children and youth. *Acta Paediatr. Scand. Suppl.*, 283:101-105, 1979.

24. Eriksson, B.O. Physical training, oxygen supply and muscle metabolism in 11- 13-year-old boys. *Acta Physiol. Scand. Suppl.*, 384:1-48, 1972.

25. Eriksson, B.O., P.D. Gollnick, and B. Saltin. The effect of physical training on muscle enzyme activities and fiber composition in 11-year-old boys. *Acta Paediatr. Belgica 28*, (suppl.):245-252, 1974.

26. Forbes, G.B. "Body composition in adolescence." In *Human growth, Vol. 2 Postnatal growth*, edited by F. Falkner and J.M. Tanner, pp. 239-272. New York: Plenum Press, 1978.

27. Fournier, M., J. Ricci, A.W. Taylor, R.J. Ferguson, R.R. Montpetit, and B.R. Chairman. Skeletal muscle adaptation in adolescent boys: Sprint and endurance training and detraining. *Med. Sci. Sports Exer.*, 14:453-456, 1982.

28. Fox, E.L. Physical training: Methods and effects. *Orthop. Clin. N. Amer.*, 8:533-548, 1977.

29. Frisch, R.E. Fatness of girls from menarche to age 18 years, with a nomogram. *Human Biol.*, 48:353-359, 1976.

30. Frisch, R.E., A.V. Gotz-Welbergen, J.W. McArthur, T. Albright, J. Witschi, B. Bullen, J. Birnholz, R.B. Reed, and H. Hermann. Delayed menarche and amenorrhea of college athletes in relation to age of onset of training. *J. Amer. Med. Assoc.*, 246:1559-1563, 1981.

31. Goldberg, A.L., J.D. Etlinger, D.F. Goldspink, and C. Jablecki. Mechanism of work-induced hypertrophy of skeletal muscle. *Med. Sci. Sports*, 7:248-261, 1975.

32. Goldspink, G. The combined effect of exercise and reduced food intake on skeletal muscle. *J. Cell. Comp. Physiol.*, 63:209-219, 1964.

33. Gollnick, P.D., R.B. Armstrong, B. Saltin, C.W. Saubert, W.L. Sembrowich, and R.E. Shepherd. Effect of training on enzyme activity and fiber composition of human skeletal muscle. *J. Appl. Physiol.*, 34:107-111, 1973.

34. Gonyea, W.J. "Muscle fiber splitting in trained and untrained animals." In *Exercise and sport science reviews* (Vol. 8), edited by R.S. Hutten and D.I. Miller, pp. 19-39. Philadelphia: Franklin Institute Press, 1980.

35. Helander, E.A.S. Influence of exercise and restricted activity on the protein composition of skeletal muscle. *Biochem. J.*, 78:478-482, 1961.

36. Holloszy, J.O. Biochemical adaptations in muscle: Effects of exercise on mitochondrial oxygen uptake and respiratory enzyme activity in skeletal muscle. *J. Biol. Chem.*, 242:2278-2282, 1967.

37. Holmer, I., and P.-O. Åstrand. Swimming training and maximal oxygen uptake. *J. Appl. Physiol.*, 33:510-513, 1972.

38. Howald, H. Ultrastructure and biochemical function of skeletal muscle in twins. *Ann. Hum. Biol.*, 3:455-462, 1976.

39. Hubbard, R.W., J.A. Smoake, W.T. Matther, J.D. Linduska, and W.S. Bowers. The effects of growth and endurance training on the protein and DNA content of rat soleus, plantaris, and gastrocnemius muscles. *Growth*, 38:171-185, 1974.

40. Huddleston, A.L., D. Rockwell, D.N. Kulund, and R.B. Harrison. Bone mass in lifetime tennis athletes. *J. Amer. Med. Assoc.*, 244:1107-1109, 1980.

41. Ilmarinen, J., and J. Rutenfranz. "Longitudinal studies of the changes in habitual activity of school children and working adolescents." In *Children and exercise IX*, edited by K. Berg and B.O. Eriksson, pp. 149-159. Baltimore: University Park Press, 1980.

42. Johnston, F.E., A.F. Roche, L.M. Schell, and N.B. Wettenhall. Critical weight at menarche: Critique of a hypothesis. *Amer. J. Dis. Child.*, 129:19-23, 1975.

43. Jones, H.H., J.D. Priest, W.C. Hayes, C.C. Tichenor, and D.H. Nagel. Humeral hypertrophy in response to exercise. *J. Bone Jt. Surg.*, 59A:204-208, 1977.

44. Kato, S., and T. Ishiko. "Obstructed growth of children's bones due to excessive labor in remote corners." In *Proceedings of international congress of sport sciences*, edited by K. Kato, p. 479. Tokyo: Japanese Union of Sport Sciences, 1966.

45. Kiiskinen, A. Physical training and connective tissues in young mice—physical properties of Achilles tendons and long bones. *Growth*, 41:123-137, 1977.

46. King, J.W., J.H. Brelsford, and H.S. Tullos. Analysis of the pitching arm of the professional baseball pitcher. *Clin. Orthop.*, 67:116-123, 1969.

47. King, D.W., and R.G. Pengelly. Effect of running exercise on the density of rat tibias. *Med. Sci. Sports*, 5:68-69, 1973.

48. Kirtland, J., and M.I. Gurr. Adipose tissue cellularity: A review. The relationship between cellularity and obesity. *Int. J. Obesity*, 3:15-55, 1979.

49. Knittle, J.L. "Adipose tissue development in man." In *Human growth, Vol. 2 Postnatal growth*, edited by F. Falkner and J.M. Tanner, pp. 295-315. New York: Plenum Press, 1978.

50. Kotulán, J., M. Reznickova, and Z. Placheta. "Exercise and growth." In *Youth and physical activity*, edited by Z. Placheta, pp. 61-117. Brno: J.E. Purkyne University Medical Faculty, 1980.

51. Krotkiewski, M., A. Aniansson, G. Grimby, P. Björntorp, and L. Sjöstrom. The effect of unilateral isokinetic strength training on local

adipose and muscle tissue morphology, thickness and enzymes. *Eur. J. Appl. Physiol.,* 42:271-281, 1979.

52. Lamb, D.R., W.D. Van Huss, R.E. Carrow, W.W. Heusner, J.C. Weber, and R. Kertzer. Effects of prepubertal physical training on growth, voluntary exercise, cholesterol and basal metabolism in rats. *Res. Quart.,* 40:123-133, 1969.

53. Lavoie, J.-M., A.W. Taylor, and R.R. Montpetit. Skeletal muscle fibre size adaptation to an eight-week swimming programme. *Eur. J. Appl. Physiol.,* 44:161-165, 1980.

54. Lopez, R., and D.M. Pruett. The child runner. *J. Phys. Educ. Rec. Dance,* 53:78-81, 1982.

55. Malina, R.M. Exercise as an influence upon growth. *Clin. Pediatr.,* 8:16-26, 1969.

56. Malina, R.M. "Anthropometric correlates of strength and motor performance." In *Exercise and sport science reviews* (Vol. 3), edited by J.H. Wilmore and J.F. Keogh, pp. 249-274. New York: Academic Press, 1975.

57. Malina, R.M. Adolescent growth and maturation: Selected aspects of current research. *Yrbk. Phys. Anthropol.,* 21:63-94, 1978.

58. Malina, R.M. "Growth of muscle tissue and muscle mass." In *Human growth, Vol. 2 Postnatal growth,* edited by F. Falkner and J.M. Tanner, pp. 273-294. New York: Plenum Press, 1978.

59. Malina, R.M. The effects of exercise on specific tissues, dimension, and functions during growth. *Studies Phys. Anthropol.,* (Wroclaw) 5:21-52, 1979.

60. Malina, R.M. "The measurement of body composition." In *Human physical growth and maturation,* edited by F.E. Johnston, A.F. Roche, and C. Susanne, pp. 35-39. New York: Plenum Press, 1980.

61. Malina, R.M. "Physical activity, growth, and functional capacity." In *Human physical growth and maturation,* edited by F.E. Johnston, A.F. Roche, and C. Susanne, pp. 303-327. New York: Plenum Press, 1980.

62. Malina, R.M. "Physical growth and maturity characteristics of young athletes." In *Children in sport* (2nd ed.), edited by R.A. Magill, M.J. Ash, and F.L. Smoll, pp. 73-96. Champaign, IL: Human Kinetics, 1982.

63. Malina, R.M. Menarche in athletes: A synthesis and hypothesis. *Ann. Human Biol.,* 10:1-24, 1983.

64. Malina, R.M., B.W. Meleski, and R. Shoup. Anthropometric, body composition and maturity characteristics of selected school-aged athletes. *Pediatr. Clin. N. Amer.,* 29:1305-1323, 1982.

65. Malina, R.M., and G.L. Rarick. "Growth, physique and motor performance." In *Physical activity: Human growth and development,* edited by G.L. Rarick, pp. 125-153. New York: Academic Press, 1973.

66. McCafferty, W.B., and S.M. Horvath. Specificity of exercise and

specificity of training: A subcellular review. *Res. Quart.*, 48:358-371, 1977.

67. Meleski, B.W., and R.M. Malina. Growth and body composition of age group swimmers 8 to 18 years of age. (In preparation.)

68. Meleski, B.W., R.F. Shoup, and R.M. Malina. Size, physique, and body composition of competitive female swimmers 11 through 20 years of age. *Human Biol.*, 54:609-625, 1982.

69. Milicer, H., and L. Denisiuk. "The physical development of youth." In *International research in sport and physical education*, edited by E. Jokl and E. Simon, pp. 262-285. Springfield, IL: Thomas, 1964.

70. Nilsson, B.E., and N.E. Westlin. Bone density in athletes. *Clin. Orthop.*, 77:179-182, 1971.

71. Novotny, V. Veranderungen des knochenalters im verlauf einer mehrjährigen sportlichen belastung. *Med. u. Sport,* 21:44-47, 1981.

72. Oscai, L.B., S.P. Babirak, J.A. McGarr, and C.N. Spirakis. Effect of exercise on adipose tissue cellularity. *Fed. Proc.*, 33:1956-1958, 1974.

73. Oscai, L.B., C.N. Spirakis, C.H. Wolff, and R.J. Beck. Effects of exercise and of food restriction on adipose tissue cellularity. *J. Lip. Res.*, 13:588-592, 1972.

74. Pařizkova, J. *Body fat and physical fitness.* The Hague: Martinus Nijhoff, 1977.

75. Pařizkova, J., and J.E.L. Carter. Influence of physical activity on stability of somatotypes in boys. *Amer. J. Phys. Anthropol.*, 44:327-339, 1976.

76. Rarick, G.L. "Competitive sports in childhood and early adolescence." In *Children in sport*, edited by R.A. Magill, M.J. Ash, and F.L. Smoll, pp. 113-128. Champaign, IL: Human Kinetics, 1978.

77. Renson, R., G. Beunen, M. Ostyn, J. Simons, J. Uytterbrouck, D. Van Gerven, and B. Van Reusel. Differentiation of physical fitness in function of sport participation. *Hermes,* (Leuven) 15:435-444, 1981.

78. Renson, R., R.M. Malina, G. Beunen, M. Ostyn, J. Simons, J. Uytterbrouck, D. Van Gerven, and B. Van Reusel. Sports participation and the growth, maturity and motor fitness of Belgian boys 12-18 years of age. (In preparation.)

79. Roche, A.F. The adipocyte-number hypothesis. *Child Dev.*, 52:31-43, 1981.

80. Rowe, F.A. Growth comparisons of athletes and non-athletes. *Res. Quart.*, 4:108-116, 1933.

81. Ruffer, W.A. A study of extreme physical activity groups of young men. *Res. Quart.*, 36:183-196, 1965.

82. Saltin, B., and L.B. Rowell. Functional adaptations to physical activity and inactivity. *Fed. Proc.*, 39:1506-1513, 1980.

83. Saville, P.D., and R. Smith. Bone density, breaking force and leg

muscle mass as functions of weight in bipedal rats. *Amer. J. Phys. Anthropol.*, 25:35-39, 1966.

84. Saville, P.D., and M.P. Whyte. Muscle and bone hypertrophy: Positive effect of running exercise in the rat. *Clin. Orthop.*, 65:81-88, 1969.

85. Scheuer, J., and C.M. Tipton. Cardiovascular adaptations to physical training. *Ann. Rev. Physiol.*, 39:221-251, 1977.

86. Schwartz, L., R.H. Britten, and L.R. Thompson. Studies in physical development and posture. 1. The effect of exercise on the physical condition and development of adolescent boys. *Pub. Health Bull.*, 179:1-38, 1928.

87. Seefeldt, V., and D. Gould. *Physical and psychological effects of athletic competition on children and youth.* ERIC Clearinghouse on Teacher Education, Washington, DC: ERIC Document No. ED 180 997, 1980.

88. Shephard, R.J., and K.H. Sidney. "Effects of physical exercise on plasma growth hormone and cortisol levels in human subjects." In *Exercise and sport science reviews* (Vol. 3), edited by J.H. Wilmore and J.F. Keogh, pp. 1-30. New York: Academic Press, 1975.

89. Steinhaus, A.H. Chronic effects of exercise. *Physiol. Rev.*, 13:103-147, 1933.

90. Tanner, J.M. *Growth at adolescence* (2nd ed.). Oxford: Blackwell, 1962.

91. Thorstensson, A. Muscle strength, fibre types and enzyme activities in man. *Acta Physiol. Scand. Suppl.*, 443:1-45, 1976.

92. Tipton, C.M., R.D. Matthes, and J.A. Maynard. Influence of chronic exercise on rat bones. *Med. Sci. Sports*, 4:55, 1972.

93. Trussell, J. Statistical flaws in evidence for the Frisch hypothesis that fatness triggers menarche. *Human Biol.*, 52:711-720, 1980.

94. Tullos, H.S., and J.W. King. Lesions of the pitching arm in adolescents. *J. Amer. Med. Assoc.*, 220:264-271, 1972.

95. Von Dobëln, W., and B.O. Eriksson. Physical training, maximal oxygen uptake and dimensions of the oxygen transporting and metabolizing organs in boys 11-13 years of age. *Acta Paediatr. Scand.*, 61:653-660, 1972.

96. Viteri, F.E., and B. Torun. "Nutrition, physical activity, and growth." In *The biology of normal human growth*, edited by M. Ritzen, A. Aperia, K. Hall, A. Larsson, A. Zetterberg, and R. Zetterström, pp. 265-273. New York: Raven Press, 1981.

97. Watson, R.C. *Bone growth and physical activity in young males.* Unpublished doctoral dissertation, University of Wisconsin, Madison, 1973.

98. Weber, G., W. Kartodihardjo, and V. Klissouras. Growth and physical training with reference to heredity. *J. Appl. Physiol.*, 40:211-215, 1976.

99. Wilmore, J.H., R.N. Girandola, and D.L. Moody. Validity of skinfold and girth assessment for predicting alterations in body composition. *J. Appl. Physiol.*, 29:313-317, 1970.

4

The Development of the Cardiorespiratory System With Growth and Physical Activity

David A. Cunningham, Donald H. Paterson,
and Cameron J.R. Blimkie
University of Western Ontario

The development of the cardiorespiratory system as children grow and take part in physical activity has been described in numerous cross-sectional but relatively few longitudinal studies, most of which have been completed in the past 10 years. The problems encountered in these studies include the difficulties of collecting data on a group of children over an extended period of time and interpreting the results in which several variables are changing simultaneously, that is, body size as well as functional capacity.

Children experience several periods of growth as they develop to adult size. During the pubescent growth spurt (lasting about 2 years), a significant portion of the growth toward adult size is attained. A peak in growth velocity is usually attained in boys at 13.5 to 14 years of age and in girls at 11.5 to 12 years of age. However the large variability in the age and magnitude of the growth spurt among different individuals imposes a difficulty in studying the functional characteristics, such as the cardiorespiratory system, in relation to growth. Chronological age-based data may therefore not be representative of true growth-related changes. If the changes in the cardiorespiratory system are also to be related to patterns of physical activity during this period of growth and development, intercorrelations between the separate factors makes the interpretation of results difficult at best, in light of the multiple variables to be studied. Such considerations require that studies involving children be carefully designed to account for the interactions of the multiple variables. Multivariate analysis, in which several variables can be held constant while the influence of a single variable is studied, has proven to be a useful tool in the study of the growth of the cardiorespiratory system with age and activity. Nevertheless, use of these statistical procedures requires relatively large subject samples followed longitudinally.

This review deals with the development of the cardiorespiratory system in growing active children, as opposed to the description of a static system at a given size or chronological age. Several reviews in the past have described the age-related changes in the cardiorespiratory system (22,38,81). This research analysis will avoid direct age-related comparison and will focus instead upon growth, maturation, and physical activity patterns in association with the development of the cardiorespiratory system.

Unfortunately, most of the functional data on the growth of the cardiorespiratory system has been collected on young boys alone. Few studies report on the development of this system in young girls. In addition, reports of several of the longitudinal studies conducted over the past decade have just begun to appear in refereed journals. The next few years should see a large increase in the information available from such longitudinal studies as the Belgian Louvain Boys Growth Study (13), the Canadian studies in Trois-Rivières (82), Saskatchewan (9), and London, Ontario (24) and a collaborative study of Norwegian and West German children (76).

METHODS FOR MEASURING
THE CARDIORESPIRATORY SYSTEM IN CHILDREN

In the studies of the cardiorespiratory response to exercise in children many of the methods have been adopted from standard protocols used in investigations of adult populations. In many cases the procedures have not been tested for validity, reliability, or reproducibility in children.

Measures of Maximum Exercise Capacity in Children

Maximal oxygen uptake ($\dot{V}O_2$ max) in children has been shown to have a reliability and reproducibility similar to that observed in adults, despite failure to always achieve a plateau in oxygen uptake. In a study of 66 10-year-old boys measured on a treadmill twice over a 4- to 5-month period, maximum heart rate and oxygen uptake were similar whether a plateau was reached or not. Boys who reached a plateau developed a larger amount of energy anaerobically, as shown by a higher post-exercise lactic acid and respiratory exchange ratio [27]. In eight 10- to 12-year-old boys who performed three repeated tests on a jog or run treadmill protocol, the coefficient of variation for $\dot{V}O_2$ max was 3 to 5%, and the reliability coefficient averaged 0.90. It was noted, however, that a walking protocol in children elicited a lower $\dot{V}O_2$ max at exhaustion, poorer reliability (0.56), and a high coefficient of variation (8%) [70]. Comparable results for $\dot{V}O_2$ max have been obtained with continuous graded treadmill protocols compared with discontinuous tests in children [84].

The use of prediction equations for estimating maximal oxygen uptake in children can be criticized on several bases. The equations most commonly used [6] were derived on an adult population and, as such, make several incorrect assumptions when applied to children. The maximal heart rates in children are often much higher than in adults with a much greater range. Further, submaximal heart rate has a relationship with height as shown by Godfrey [38]; heart rate at a given power output was one beat per minute lower for each centimeter of height increase (range 100-180 cm). To illustrate the problem of prediction from submaximal tests, it has been shown that weight and fatness alone can account for the major variance in $\dot{V}O_2$max among children of similar age (cumulative $R^2 = .77$) [25]. Thus, in this case the taller children have lower submaximal heart rates at a given power output and the heavier children have larger values for $\dot{V}O_2$max. Direct studies comparing predicted with measured maximal values have found an average error as large as 20% [43,88].

The use of submaximal tests, such as the PWC_{170}, to describe maximal working capacity is not appropriate. In this, as in adult studies, a proper maximal test is needed to find $\dot{V}O_2$max. The test may be useful as a relative score of fitness and has been used in several population surveys for this purpose. In this case, however, a further error may be made if comparisons are made across different age groups or across different maturational ages, or in fact among subjects of the same age but different body size. The only possible use may be in describing the average values for a population at a specific age. The range in this case would be very great and lead to possible misinterpretation in comparison studies.

Measures of Cardiorespiratory Function in Children

Cardiac output, stroke volume, and arterial-venous oxygen difference have been measured by direct determination (dye dilution) in only a few cases in children (21,32). The CO_2 rebreathing technique has been successfully utilized for the determination of exercise cardiac output in children (10,35,40,69,100). Paterson et al. (72) found that exercise cardiac output measures had a day-to-day coefficient of variation of 7 to 8% compared to adult values of 4 to 7%. The larger variability of $\dot{Q}$ in children compared with adults was accounted for in part by greater biological changes in the submaximal exercise response as illustrated by the simple measures of heart rate in which children had a variability of 4 to 6% compared to 2 to 3% in adults. The greatest source of variation apparently lies in the estimation of arterial CO_2 tension. Nevertheless, the CO_2 rebreathing technique provides a reliable noninvasive method for estimating the cardiac output in exercise, and as such is an important tool in assessing the cardiorespiratory system of children.

Methods of Data Analysis Particular to Children

In several recent studies (24,66) the growth of the cardiorespiratory system has been modeled on a mathematical system. Changes over chronological ages and maturative ages have been described as growth functions with the use of computer assisted curve-fitting routines (1,73). These techniques have greatly simplified the problems of describing growth patterns with longitudinal data.

GROWTH AND THE DEVELOPMENT
OF THE CARDIORESPIRATORY SYSTEM

The interaction between normal growth, physical activity, and the development of the cardiorespiratory system in children has been frequently studied and Godfrey (39) has presented an extensive review. Many of these studies are cross-sectional (3,16,25,35,42), and chronological age rather than level of maturation is used as the reference factor. In such instances, differences attributed to age or body size are confounded by the wide variation in maturation, and growth-specific influences on the cardiorespiratory system are hidden. Some of the recently published longitudinal studies (54,66,86) have presented an analysis of the influence of growth and maturation on the cardiorespiratory system, rather than simply the static relationship with body size and age.

Cross-sectional studies have described the submaximal exercise cardio-respiratory response of children. Generally, the level of oxygen uptake and cardiac output during submaximal exercise is dependent upon work rate and independent of body size (32,35,38,42). However, stroke volume is dependent upon body size and is therefore related to age (35,40,42,78). Figure 4-1 illustrates this relationship developed from longitudinal data (24). In addition, the arterial-venous oxygen difference $(a - \bar{v}O_2$ diff) at a given workrate appears dependent upon age and/or body size. These differences in arterial-venous oxygen extraction were due to the slightly greater efficiency (lower $\dot{V}O_2$ at a given workrate) in the older boys. In heavy work the highest $a - \bar{v}O_2$ difference was constant across ages.

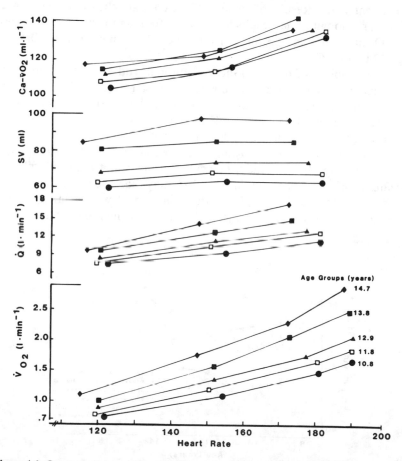

Figure 4-1. Oxygen uptake, cardiac output, stroke volume, and arterial-venous oxygen difference against work rates on a cycle ergometer in 62 boys studied longitudinally at ages 10.8, 12.9, and 14.7 years (24).

Maximal Oxygen Uptake

The effect of maximal exercise on the cardiorespiratory system has been reported in several cross-sectional studies (37,67,97,100). Maximal oxygen uptake (l • min^{-1}) is larger in older children, but when weight is used as a reference factor (ml • kg^{-1} • min^{-1}) this relationship is not always evident. Studies have shown variable findings in this area; no change, a slight increase, or a decline with age in $\dot{V}O_2$max per kilogram of body weight. This discrepancy in the results may be due to the cross-sectional nature of the data and the differences in the samples of children studied. Similar results have been found in longitudinal studies with boys. When maximal oxygen uptake is divided by body weight the values increase (24,54), decrease (7,76—German boys only) or stay approximately constant with age (76—Norwegian boys, 86) from pre- to post-pubescent years. Results of some of these data are shown in Figure 4-2. With girls, longitudinal results have most often demonstrated a decrease in $\dot{V}O_2$max (ml • kg^{-1} • min^{-1}) with age. This is most evident beyond age 12 to 13 (76).

The variability of results in the longitudinal studies may be due to the fact that weight per se is not always the best reference factor for the growth of the cardiorespiratory system in this range. In a study in which 81 boys were tested annually from age 10 to 15 (24), the relationship of weight with $\dot{V}O_2$max showed a different level of importance at each age. The explained variance in $\dot{V}O_2$max due to weight ranged from 50 to 70% in ages 9 to 15. In this study, however, weight was found to explain a greater proportion of the variance in $\dot{V}O_2$max than the other size factors such as height and fatness. Thus, the influence of weight in explaining the variance in $\dot{V}O_2$ among subjects fluctuates during the growth years of

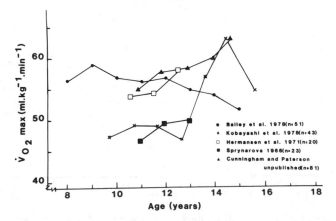

Figure 4-2. Maximal oxygen uptake (ml • kg^{-1} • min^{-1}) on the treadmill from longitudinal studies of boys ranging in age from 8 to 16 years (data adapted from published reports).

9 to 15. The weight changes during this period in relation to the changes in cardiorespiratory function, however, are not as important in describing individual development. The relationship between weight and function at individual ages may be fortuitous and could result from a large variation in weight among the children at any age.

Other dimensional components based on height have been suggested as reference factors to standardize the relationship of $\dot{V}O_2$ with size (4,64,96). In longitudinal observations of $\dot{V}O_2max$ in boys, the exponent of height 2.46 was found to best describe the actual relationship of age to $\dot{V}O_2max$. This closely approximates the 2.5 exponent for height which is analogous to Kleiber's (51) three-fourth power of body weight as the best theoretical representation of metabolic body size (8). Davies et al. (29) have shown leg volume to provide a close relationship with $\dot{V}O_2max$. Leg volume explained sex and age differences in $\dot{V}O_2max$ and accounted for over 80% of the variance in $\dot{V}O_2max$. However, Ross et al. (75) have emphasized that boys do not sustain a similar shape and body composition at all ages. A single size adjustment is inadequate to express relative metabolic functional values. Various body size component factors may be needed to explain the growth of the cardiorespiratory function during the years around puberty. Additional longitudinal studies are needed, therefore, in order to explore the proportionality of functional aspects with growth characteristics.

Cardiac Output and Arterial-Venous Oxygen Difference

Several cross-sectional studies have reported measures of cardiac output, stroke volume, and arterial-venous oxygen difference during near maximum exercise in children of different ages. Results from a number of these cross-sectional studies suggest that cardiac output and stroke volume increase with age and growth throughout childhood and adolescence (37,38,67,97,100). In addition, at a specific chronological age the variability of $\dot{V}O_2$ is explained largely by the differences in stroke volume (58 to 78% of the variance) (24).

Stroke volume is determined to a significant extent by body size in children ages 12 to 14 years. In a study of 117 boys age 9 to 15, subjects with a large maximum oxygen uptake were found to have significantly larger (echocardiographic) internal cardiac dimensions (left ventricular end diastolic diameter and left ventricular mass) and resting cardiac function (stroke volume). Thus, the larger stroke volume of subjects with larger aerobic power was attributed to significantly larger left ventricular end diastolic diameters and volumes. The strong relation between cardiac dimensions and stroke volume, as well as $\dot{V}O_2max$, was mainly attributed to the shared influence of body size on both these factors (15).

Arterial-venous oxygen difference has been observed to be larger in older children (67). Weber et al. (97) and Gilliam et al. (37) found a steady increase in $a - \bar{v}O_2$ difference across ages 10 to 13, whereas Yamaji and Miyashita (100) did not observe a consistent trend in this age range. Beyond age 13 little increase was found in this variable (97,100). The maximal $a - \bar{v}O_2$ difference in prepubertal children is less than that found in adults (40) and, based on cross-sectional studies, seems to increase slightly with age during childhood, eventually approaching adult values in late adolescence.

It is evident that there is substantial development of cardiorespiratory functions and maximal oxygen uptake in children as they increase in age and body size. It is not known whether the capacity of the cardiorespiratoy system increases at a constant rate during the prepubertal, pubertal, and postpubertal stages of development in children or whether there is preferential development of the stroke volume (heart size and function) or arterial-venous oxygen difference (oxygen delivery or utilization) at different stages of growth and development which account for these observed changes. These questions cannot be answered using a cross-sectional approach. Longitudinal studies that follow children through puberty and simultaneously evaluate the development of the cardiorespiratory system are required to solve these problems.

PHYSICAL ACTIVITY AND THE DEVELOPMENT OF THE CARDIORESPIRATORY SYSTEM

The study of the influence of physical activity or exercise training upon the development of the cardiorespiratory system in children is confounded by several important normally occurring factors in this age range: (a) the age- and size-related changes in this physiologic system; (b) the natural propensity of physical activity among healthy children; and (c) the heterogeneity of physical maturation at chronological ages near puberty, which will result in comparisons being made between children of similar chronological but different maturative ages. Most studies have failed to account for all of these problems and, for this reason, much of the past research has produced results from which it is difficult to draw firm conclusions.

Implications Regarding Physical Activity From Study of Athletic Children

A number of studies have attempted to indicate the effects of physical activity by comparing the cardiorespiratory responses of athletic to nonathletic children or normative data. Children who participate in competitive sports have greater submaximal work capacity and maximal oxygen uptake values (5,23,26,44,79,98) than the nonactive reference groups. Two studies by Andrew et al. (3) and Hamilton and Andrew (42) have compared stroke volume during submaximal exercise in athletic and nonathletic groups. Lower heart rate but similar stroke volume was found in trained swimmers, and prepubertal ice-hockey players showed no difference in heart rate or stroke volume compared to the reference samples. Sports participation prior to the pubertal growth spurt may thus have little effect on the cardiorespiratory system in contrast to observations in adolescents.

The major problem in these study designs may be the confounding effect of different maturation levels; for boys, the athletic groups usually are of a select nature and tend to be advanced in biological maturity (61). In addition, it could be suggested that the more mature boy with greater skill development may be more active in everyday activities aside from the involvement in organized athletics.

Physical Activity Assessment in Children

In order to account for the effect of regular activity levels in studies comparing different groups of children (athlete vs. nonathlete or training group vs. control), there is need for a sensitive, simple, and valid measurement tool of physical activity. The difficulty in developing such a tool is illustrated by the number of techniques that have been tried and found wanting. In 28 boys (age 12) daily energy expenditure was determined by heart rate and stepping frequencies recorded on an Oxford Medilog tape recorder for several days, and participation in regular physical activity was determined by a questionnaire concerning the number of activity pursuits engaged in over the previous year. In a multivariate design, body mass and fatness made the only significant contributions to the variance in $\dot{V}O_2$max ($R^2 = .77$). Measures of daily energy expenditure, the time the heart rate was above a training threshold, and number of regular physical activities added little to the explained variance ($R^2 = .78$), (25). Questionnaires of daily physical activity do not appear to be sensitive to the small differences in activity levels among normal children.

Gilliam et al. (36) have also used the Oxford system for Holter monitoring in prepubescent children (22 boys, 18 girls) ages 6 to 7. Heart rates exceeding 160 beats $\cdot$ min^{-1} occurred 21 min and 9 min for boys and girls, respectively, during the 12-hour monitoring period. The authors concluded that although the children appeared moderately active, they seldom experienced high intensity physical activity. Boys in this sample were involved in more vigorous activities than the girls. This method of determining activity levels is much more specific, but is limited to the study of small groups due to the considerable time involved.

Kemper and Verschuur (48) investigated the uses of hip pedometers in 30 boys (ages 12-18). They found that the actual rate of stepping on a treadmill and that measured with a pedometer were very different, the errors being greatest at slow speeds. At speeds of 6, 8, and 10 km • h^{-1}, the error was approximately 3%. Running at 14 km • h^{-1} gave an overestimation of about 8.5%. At 2 km • h^{-1} the underestimation was about 70%. This technique appears to have limited use with children, although the overall error apparently gives a conservative estimate of the actual activity level.

In order to describe the daily energy expenditure, caloric intake was determined through a 24-hour recall questionnaire and interview of the boys and their parents in a study by Thompson et al. (94). The caloric value of the foods eaten was determined from approximations using food models of quantity, and energy intake was calculated from standard tables. The results indicated that the 104 boys (ages 10 to 14) involved in highly active competitive ice hockey teams, or age-matched controls in less active recreational pursuits, did not differ in their daily caloric intake per kilogram of body weight (73 vs. 68 kilocalories per kilogram). Caloric intake based on daily energy needs appeared to be determined by general levels of childhood activities rather than the briefer periods of organized sport, as assumed in comparisons of athletic and nonathletic children.

Mirwald et al. (66) have made a rigorous attempt to classify children's physical activity through yearly ratings by teachers and parents and interviews with the children. The validity of this method has not been reported. The results of simple questionnaires have been studied in a multivariate design, and when size factors are accounted for, activity habits have not been related to cardiorespiratory fitness in children (15,25). Physical activity profiles add little to the explained variance in cardiorespiratory fitness of children.

Table 4-1

Study	Sex	Age	No.	Training Wks	Type of Training
Brown et al. (1972)	F	8-13	12	6 12	Continuous running, interval training, pursuit games
Von Dobeln & Eriksson (1972)	M	11-13	12	16	Running for speed, time, & distance, cross-country skiing & gymnastics
Koch & Eriksson (1973)	M	11-13	9	16	High-speed interval running, cross-country skiing

Short-Term Training and Development
of the Cardiorespiratory System

Studies of the effect of short-term training programs (less than 6 months) on the cardiorespiratory system have been reviewed in earlier publications (8,22,61). Selected data are summarized in Table 4-1. While the majority of these studies have reported significant increases in $\dot{V}O_2$max, maximal work capacity, or reduction in submaximal heart rate in either boys or girls (19,33,56,60,63,80,89,95,96,97), a few studies reported no change in these variables (11,47,68). Lack of improvement may be attributed to the athletic involvement of the subjects prior to the training program per se (47), or to the maturative age of the children (prepubescent) (11,77). In these cases the training program adds very little to the already very active daily recreational pursuits of the children. It has been impossible, from the studies demonstrating an improvement in cardiorespiratory fitness, to assess the actual intensity of the training stimuli needed to promote this change. It is also possible that programs of interval type training have not been as effective as regimens emphasizing continuous training.

Studies have also been carried out with exercise programs in a regular school physical education class. Goode et al. (41) found that over a 4-month period, with the addition of 6 min daily, of large muscle physical activities (skipping, running, hopping) eliciting heart rates between 150-165 beats $\cdot$ min^{-1}, the aerobic power was significantly increased in boys ages 12 to 14 and girls ages 12 and 14, but not in 13-year-old girls. Bar-Or and Zwiren (11) found that increased frequency of physical education classes for 9- and 10-year-old boys and girls resulted in no significant improvement in cardiorespiratory fitness. Kemper et al. (50)

Summary of Short-Term (<6 Months) Training Studies in Children

Intensity of Training	$\dot{V}O_2$ or PWC max	SV submax	SV max
1-2 hrs/day 4-5 times/wk	Sign*		
3 times/wk, for 1 hr	Sign		
3 times/wk for 1 hr, 15 sec to 5 min exercise intervals	Sign		Sign

Table 4-1 (Cont.)

Study	Sex	Age	No.	Training Wks	Type of Training
Eriksson & Koch (1973)	M	11	5	16	High-speed running, vigorous gymnastics, cross-country skiing
Eriksson et al. (1974)	M	11	5	6	Endurance training 20-30 min/day, 3 times/wk
Bar-Or & Zwiren (1973)	M F	9-10 9-10	48 48	9 9	Phys. ed. classes & endurance interval runs
Mocellin & Wasmund (1973)	M F	7.6 to 10.3	53	6-7	Running training
Massicotte & MacNab (1974)	M	11-13	36	6	Cycle training
Stewart & Gutin (1976)	M	10-12	24	8	Interval running, & all out work
Weber et al. (1976)	M	10, 13, 16	24	10	Distance running, continuous step work, intermittent cycling
Lussier & Buskirk (1977)	M F	8-12 8-12	20 6	12 12	Continuous running, running games & activities
Kellet et al. (1978)	M F	15-16 15-16	6 9	12 12	Swim training
Vanfraechem & Vanfraechem-Raway (1978)	F	12-14	20	16	Endurance activities, speed, litheness, & strength

*Sign—indicates a significant increase ($p < 0.05$)
Adapted from Blimkie (14)

Summary of Short-Term (<6 Months) Training Studies in Children (Cont.)

Intensity of Training	$\dot{V}O_2$ or PWC max	SV submax	SV max
3 times/wk for 1 hr, 85-90% $\dot{V}O_2$max	Sign	Sign at 250, 500, and 750 kpm•min^{-1}	Sign
70-85% $\dot{V}O_2$max	Sign		
Regular class plus 2, 3, or 4 sessions/ wk for 20-25 min/day	No change No change		
Max speed over 1000m, twice/wk or 800 m, once/wk, 94-95% $\dot{V}O_2$max	No change No change		
130-140, 150-160, 170-180 b•min^{-1}, 3 times/wk for 12 min	Sign PWC all groups sign $\dot{V}O_2$max in 170-180 b•min^{-1} group only		
90% HR max, 1 min runs over 250 yd, 3-min paced runs over 600 yd	No change		
1 mi, max effort HR around 162 b•min^{-1} for 8.5 min, 3 min bouts at HR max, until exhausted	No change In 13-yr-olds, sign $\dot{V}O_2$max in 10- & 16-yr-olds	No change in 13-yr olds, sign in 10- & 16-yr-olds	
75-80% $\dot{V}O_2$max, 2-5 times/wk, for 10-35 min	No changes in absolute $\dot{V}O_2$max sign in relative $\dot{V}O_2$max		
6000m/session 8 times/wk	Sign		
HR 150•min^{-1}, 3 times/ wk for 1-1½ hrs	No change Sign in pred. $\dot{V}O_2$max		

showed no improvement in 12- and 13-year-old boys. Shephard et al. (82) have reported the preliminary cross-sectional results of an ongoing longitudinal program in Trois-Rivières, Canada, the purpose of the study being to describe the effect of physical activity on various parameters of growth and development between the ages of 5 and 12. The physical activity levels were increased in half the classes of two community schools (ages 6 to 11). Gains in maximal oxygen uptake and muscular strength beyond that due to growth were found in groups with the added physical education programs.

Children involved in training programs for up to 6 months have demonstrated either no change (60) or a significant increase (33,56) in stroke volume during submaximal exercise. The critical factor appears to be the age of the children in these studies. The younger children in the study by Lussier and Buskirk (60) are less likely to demonstrate the usual training effect. Eriksson and Koch (33) also show that maximal cardiac output, stroke volume, and a $-\bar{v}O_2$ difference are increased with training.

Long-Term Training and Development
of the Cardiorespiratory System

Exercise training in children that lasts longer than 6 months would be referred to as long-term in scope. The development of the cardiorespiratory system is partly a function of growth; therefore, the interpretation of an exercise training program that lasts for several months or

Table 4-2

Study	Sex	Age	No.	Training Period	Type of Training
Sprynarova (1966)	M	11-13	114	24 mo	I Athletics II Basketball III No extra school activity IV Mixed activity All Ss grouped
Ekblom (1969)	M	11-13.6	6	6 mo	I Interval training, dash training, distance running, strength training, ball games
			7	32 mo	II No extra school activity

more will be confounded by normal growth. It is not surprising that all such investigations have reported increases in the absolute $\dot{V}O_2$max (Table 4-2). Since any interpretation of research will be influenced by normal growth, all investigations of this type would require the use of a control or reference sample. Even in this case, the experimental and control groups may experience different rates of growth over the investigative period by chance alone. When study numbers are very small and truly random samples are not used, such discrepancies are more likely to occur. In addition, when the groups are self-selected based upon their early success in sports, the active group will usually represent early maturers (61). In such studies, body weight has been used as the reference factor to account for differences in growth patterns among the groups; however, Mirwald et al. (66) have pointed out that height may be the preferred standard. They state that height is known to be fitted by standard mathematical growth curves and that it is less affected by environmental factors (nutritional patterns) than is weight.

In the long-term training studies, three different models for investigation have been used: studies of comparison of athletes and nonathletes, recreational activity groups and reference groups, and specialized training programs with control subjects. None of the studies to date have actually used a random assignment to the training of control groups, a technique that would help interpret the findings but would be difficult to design in a normal community.

Studies that have reported results on training during the age range prior to and approaching puberty include the study of Swedish boys (30)

Summary of Long-Term (>6 Months) Training Studies In Children

Intensity of Training	$\dot{V}O_2$max ($L \cdot min^{-1}$)	$\dot{V}O_2$max ($ml \cdot kg^{-1} \cdot min^{-1}$)
	2.4% overall	3.6% overall
	27.98% overall	7.3% overall
	25.1% overall	4.6% overall
	28.9% overall	4.8% overall
	27.2% overall	5.0% overall
At least twice/wk averaging 6-60 min, max HR during intervals, full speed during dashes, HR 130-180 $b \cdot min^{-1}$ during distance runs	15% and 18% above controls at 6 & 32 mo	10% above controls at 6 mo, but no difference at 32 mo

Table 4-2 (Cont.)

Study	Sex	Age	No.	Training Period	Type of Training
Daniels & Oldridge (1971)	M	10-15	6	22 mo	Steady running training
Berg & Bjure (1974)	M	13	13	6-30 mo	Training for cycling races
Sprynarova (1974)	M	11-18	39	7 yrs	I Regularly trained in basketball and track & field
					II Irregularly trained in various sports
					III Untrained
Kobayashi et al. (1978)	M	9-18	56	6 yrs	I Endurance running, soccer, & swimming
				5 yrs	II No specialized training from ages 12-18
				3 yrs	III Competitive middle- & long-distance running from ages 14-17
Sprynarova et al. (1978)	M	12-15	8	3 yrs	I Swimming
	F	12-15	12	3 yrs	II Swimming
Mirwald et al. (1981)	M	7-17	25	10 yrs	I Active; high level of habitual activity and sports participation
					II Inactive; low level of habitual activity and sports participation

Adapted from Blimkie (14)

Summary of Long-Term (>6 Months) Training Studies in Children (Cont.)

Intensity of Training	$\dot{V}O_2max$ (L·min^{-1})	$\dot{V}O_2max$ (ml·kg^{-1}·min^{-1})
Between 336 to 2000 miles/yr average	21.8% overall, between 12 & 14 yrs > increase between 12.4 & 13.0 yrs	2.0% overall, between 12 & 14 yrs > increase between 12.1 & 12.4 yrs Significant for 1st 6 mo, no change afterward
At least 2 sessions for 4 or 6 hrs/wk	118.2% overall, > increase between 13-14 yrs	13.1% overall, > increase between 13-14 yrs
Irregular sessions 2 or 3 hrs/wk	98.3% overall, > increase between 13-14 yrs	5.6% overall, > increase between 13-14 yrs
1 hr/wk up to 15 yrs, no training thereafter	98.7% overall, > increase between 13-14 yrs	2.7% overall, > increase between 13-14 yrs
1-1½ hr/day, 4-5 times/wk	132.5% overall, > increase from 12.7-13.7 yrs	15.8% overall, > increase from 12.7-13.7 yrs
Regular phys. ed.	59.7% overall, > increase from 13.1-14.1 yrs	15.1% overall, > increase from 13.1-14.1 yrs
Regular middle- & long-distance running	25.4% overall	15.8% overall
11 sessions/wk, increased load each yr	57.6% overall, > increase from 14-15 yrs	10.7% overall, > increase from 14-15 yrs
11 sessions/wk, increased load each yr	31.6% overall, > increase from 12-13 yrs	10.8% overall, > increase from 14-15 yrs
No indication	250% overall, > increase from 12-14 yrs & slightly after age of PHV	
No indication	233% overall, > increase from 11-14 yrs & slightly after age of PHV	

who trained for 6 and 32 months during the age range of 11 to 13.6 years. An increase was observed in $\dot{V}O_2max$ of 15% and 18% in $1 \cdot min^{-1}$ and 10% in $ml \cdot kg^{-1} \cdot min^{-1}$ after 6 months, with no difference between the trained and control groups after 32 months. This suggests that the improvement in cardiorespiratory capacity was related to size.

This phenomenon can be illustrated with several other studies. Czechoslovakian boys who trained for athletics or basketball between age 11 to 13 showed little additional development in $\dot{V}O_2max$ $(1 \cdot min^{-1})$ beyond that attributed to growth (85,86). In Canadian boys, high and relatively low active groups between ages 11 to 13 showed no difference in the increase in $\dot{V}O_2max$ (65). Kobayashi et al. (54) found a substantial increase in $\dot{V}O_2max$ in boys trained from age 9.7 to 12.7, a change that may also be attributed to growth since a control group was not included for this subset of boys.

When boys in their pubertal growth years are studied, increases in $\dot{V}O_2max$ of trained groups compared to control groups are observed. Notwithstanding the fact that the active groups in these studies were self-selected and therefore may display different maturational rates in the growth of the cardiorespiratory system, there was an increase in $\dot{V}O_2max$ relative to body mass $(ml \cdot kg^{-1} \cdot min^{-1})$ beyond that in the reference samples (54,66,86). Mirwald et al. (66) used height as the reference factor and also observed a higher level of $\dot{V}O_2max$ during the period of greatest growth (peak height velocity). However, there remains some doubt whether these changes were significant.

Training in adolescence (14.5 to 18 y) has produced results similar to those found in adult groups. The $\dot{V}O_2max$ in $1 \cdot min^{-1}$ was increased beyond that due to growth (54,86). Kobayashi et al. (54) found a 15.8% increase in $\dot{V}O_2max$ $(ml \cdot kg^{-1} \cdot min^{-1})$ in the 3 years from ages 14 to 17.

Problems in studying exercise training during this period of growth are numerous and are obviously confounded by the heterogeneity of the growth patterns in children. The data above suggests, but does not confirm, that exercise training may have its greatest impact when begun during the period of greatest growth. The concept of a critical period, corresponding to the pubertal growth spurt, for the enhanced development of the cardiorespiratory system remains to be proved. This issue could be resolved by studying a control group of normally active boys and an experimental group exposed to a rigorous, supervised, and quantifiable exercise routine—initiated prior to the pubertal growth spurt and continued for a couple of years beyond this time. In addition, a monozygotic split twin design in which one child trains and the other serves as a control over the years of the rapid growth period may also be a useful study technique.

HEREDITY AND THE DEVELOPMENT
OF THE CARDIORESPIRATORY SYSTEM

The influence of heredity on the development of the cardiorespiratory system has been reported in several recent papers (45,52,53,57,59,97) and reviewed by Bouchard (17). Klissouras (52,53) has described the correlations for maximal aerobic power (ml $\cdot$ kg^{-1} $\cdot$ min^{-1}) in studies of twins. In these studies both monozygotic twins and dizygotic twins were tested for maximal oxygen uptake on a treadmill. The genetic factor was found to be the principle determinant of the variability in $\dot{V}O_2$max, with the hereditability estimate showing maximal oxygen uptake to be greater than 90% genetically determined. The intraclass correlations in the monozygotic (MZ) and dizygotic (DZ) twin pairs were .91 to .95 and .36 to .44, respectively. Other variables showed intraclass correlations of .84 to .90 (MZ) and .62 to .84 (DZ) for heart rate, and .60 (MZ) and .61 (DZ) for heart volume per kg of body weight. These very high values for the heredity factor have been criticized in recent years, and estimates have been set much lower. Considerably more research needs to be done with twins before the genetic contribution can be estimated in a more precise manner. A training study with twins (97) has shown that the genotype was a major determinant of work capacity since the maximal trainability of $\dot{V}O_2$max was only about 40% of the initial level. Howald (45) found that $\dot{V}O_2$max increased 15% in a trained twin (MZ) relative to the sibling. These observations suggest that vigorous athletic training cannot contribute to the maximal aerobic power beyond a limit set by the genotype. Heredity influences the development of structural and organic attributes, factors which impose limits to the development of physical fitness.

The genetic factors appear to influence the ultimate development of body size (height and weight), which in turn may account for the level of attained $\dot{V}O_2$max. Muscle fiber composition may also be set by hereditary factors and may be independent of body size (57). This again would suggest that in addition to body size, the influence of genetic factors on $\dot{V}O_2$max may operate through the genetic determination of skeletal muscle fiber type and distribution. On the other hand, both MZ and DZ twins show similar variation in their muscle enzyme activities (45,58,83). Thus although the genetic influence may be important in the development of body size and muscle fiber composition, the training factor appears to be important in the functional capacity of muscle.

The genetic contribution to the development of the cardiorespiratory system has been studied in relation to structural components such as heart size (53). The functional characteristics of the cardiorespiratory system such as stroke volume and arterial-venous oxygen difference have not been studied with the twin model. At present, little is known of the genetic influence on the functional capacity of the heart.

MATURATION AND THE DEVELOPMENT OF THE CARDIORESPIRATORY SYSTEM

Cross-sectional data have shown body size to be a significant determinant of the exercise oxygen uptake in boys ages 10 to 14. Inference of growth effects of physiological functions from cross-sectional design usually fails to account for differences in physical maturation among subjects of the same chronological age. A few such studies have attempted to account for maturation in the cross-sectional designs (26,27,49,71) using measurement of hand skeletal age. Kemper and Verschuur (49) measured $\dot{V}O_2$max in 375 boys and girls ages 13 and 14. Biological age (hand-wrist X-ray) of the sample ranged from 9 to 16 years. This study found that almost all of the variation of $\dot{V}O_2$max among (inter-subject variation) the children was due to the increase in height or mass. Biological age per se explained only an insignificant part of the total variance (less than 8%). When changes in $\dot{V}O_2$max were analyzed across biological age (intra-subject variation), controlled for chronological age, most of the explained variation was due to biological age. The relation of biological age with $\dot{V}O_2$max acted through the strong relation between biological age and body height or mass. The development of $\dot{V}O_2$max appears to be influenced by a body size maturation interaction.

The longitudinal design for the study of the influence of growth on the cardiorespiratory system has been employed by several investigators (2,7,30,43,54,66,74,76,86). These studies were limited in certain aspects. In the studies of Ekblom (30), Hermansen and Oseid (43) and Andersen et al. (2), subjects were not followed throughout the growth period. In the reports of Bailey (7), Sprynarova (86), and Rutenfranz et al. (76), data were expressed at chronological ages and thus failed to account for individual biological differences. Data of Kobayashi et al. (54) and Mirwald et al. (66) have been expressed relative to the individual's age of peak height velocity, thus standardizing maturative status (91,92) among subjects during the period of rapid physical development.

Maturative Age-Based Longitudinal Studies

The Saskatchewan Child Growth and Development Study was a 10-year (1964 through 1973) longitudinal investigation of growth (20,65,66). Some 207 7-year-old boys were randomly selected for the study on a stratified socioeconomic basis from the city elementary schools; at completion of the study 131 boys were examined. Girls (100 subjects ages 7 to 15) in a mixed longitudinal design were also added to this study, but no data have been published on them. This study measured many aspects of the boys' and girls' health and physiological responses to a treadmill exercise test. The boys' data were related to the age of peak height velocity in order to determine whether changes in aerobic power were due to normal growth and/or exercise programs. Peak height velocity, which usually occurs in boys between the ages of 13 and 14, is a common fixing or centering point for longitudinal developmental analyses. Data of chronological age-based standards for $\dot{V}O_2$max ($l \cdot min^{-1}$) and for $\dot{V}O_2$max velocity ($l \cdot min^{-1} \cdot y^{-1}$) have been published (20,65). Peak $\dot{V}O_2$max velocity at 14 years of age compared to the time of peak height velocity was slightly delayed (up to 4 months). Testosterone secretion is observed to increase about 4 months after peak height velocity and at the time of peak $\dot{V}O_2$ velocity. This relationship was thought to be related to the slight delay in peak $\dot{V}O_2$max relative to peak height velocity and has been proven a factor in the development of muscle strength, and increase in hemoglobin and red blood cells (66).

Mirwald et al. (66) assessed activity levels of 15 of the boys and determined the relationship with growth. The active boys had a greater growth of $\dot{V}O_2$max immediately following age of peak height velocity, and this increase relative to the inactive boys was extended over a much longer period of time. Adolescence was considered to be a critical period for the development of a high $\dot{V}O_2$max. It was noted that boys who have a genetic endowment for a high $\dot{V}O_2$max may have become more active at this period of growth than those with a limited genetic ceiling, and that at adolescence a widened difference in physical activities emerges.

Kobayashi et al. (54) studied seven boys ages 9 to 16 involved in endurance activities over a 5-year period, and six distance runners ages 14 to 17. An additional 43 boys were studied from 12 to 18 years and used as a reference sample. Maximal oxygen uptake was determined on a treadmill and plotted against peak height velocity. Data showed that training before the age of 12 years had little effect on aerobic power while training in the year prior to age of peak height velocity and thereafter resulted in an increased $\dot{V}O_2$max beyond that expected during the adolescent growth spurt (although the reference group was not followed up to or after the growth period). Results appear to support the hypothesis that there is a critical period for the development of $\dot{V}O_2$max related to increased physical activity at the time of rapid growth. On the other hand, the lack of differences between pubertal stages in hormone concentrations (testosterone, growth hormone, insulin) resulting from acute exercise suggests that there may not be a critical stage of enhanced response to exercise training (34).

In both of the longitudinal reports (54,66) very few subjects were studied. At best, data on these few boys (less than 15 active boys in either study) is subject to the confounding influences of differences in maturative rates between the active and inactive groups. Although aligned on peak height velocity, boys of different onset of maturation (early or late) may show markedly different cardiorespiratory responses to exercise. For example, early maturers have shown higher values for size, strength, and performance measures at a given chronological age (61). On the other hand, $\dot{V}O_2max$ for late maturers at a given maturational age prior to peak height velocity (PHV) has been found consistently higher than in normal or early maturers (24, Figure 4-3). Activity level and maturation are also related and may confound the interpretation of results. The inactive subjects in Mirwald's studies were also the later maturers based on skeletal age. The changes attributed to inactivity may also reflect differences of age of maturation.

In a study (24) of growth and development of the cardiorespiratory system, 81 boys of a total intake of 151 were followed for 4 years, ages 9.8 to 14.8. Yearly measurements were made of size and anthropometric variables, treadmill $\dot{V}O_2max$, and stroke volume and arterial-venous oxygen difference during steady-state cycle ergometry. Peak height velocity (PHV) and hand-wrist X-rays were used to describe the level of maturation in this study. When the $\dot{V}O_2max$ was related to the age at PHV, there were no large differences in the year-to-year changes in $\dot{V}O_2max$ (-1 to O PHV), (Figure 4-4).

In the same longitudinal study, stroke volume appeared to demonstrate a large increase during the year following the age of rapid growth (year of PHV $+1$). The increase in stroke volume was probably due to both structural and functional adaptations. However, Bouchard et al. (18) and Blimkie et al. (15) have indicated a decreasing heart size to body

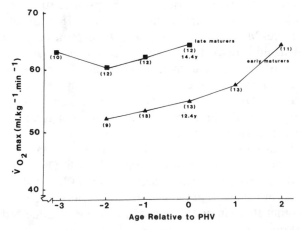

Figure 4-3. Maximal oxygen uptake (ml · kg^{-1} · min^{-1}) on the treadmill vs. maturative age in a longitudinal study. Early and late maturers were determined from skeletal age confirmed by age of peak height velocity (24).

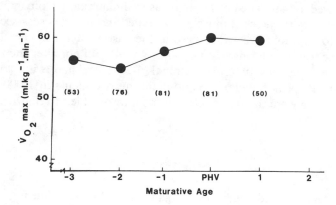

Figure 4-4. Maximum oxygen uptake (ml • kg^{-1} • min^{-1}) on the treadmill vs. maturative age in a longitudinal study of 81 boys (24). Due to different maturative rates among these boys the number of subjects at each point is reduced.

weight ratio from prepuberty to adolescence. It appears that the growth of the heart does not keep pace with somatic growth, but the increase in absolute terms may contribute to an increased stroke volume. The change in stroke volume, however, appears to be due primarily to changes in the functional capacity of the cardiorespiratory system rather than size of the heart alone. An increased preload related to increased venous return from a large active tissue mass may be important. Training in adults has shown similar changes to these changes observed in young children progressing through the developmental years (93,99). The increase in $\dot{V}O_2$ during the year preceding that of PHV is apparently related to the widened $a - \bar{v}O_2$ difference. The association of a widened $a - \bar{v}O_2$ difference with the period of most rapid growth may also be secondary to the increased muscle mass (62). This increased muscle may be accompanied by altered muscle enzymatic profiles and the capillary to fiber ratio (62). Koch (55) has described changes in regional muscle blood flow which also coincide with this period of development. Further, increased O_2 carrying capacity of the blood may depend on maturation (90).

The development of oxygen uptake capacity during the age of growth appears to be dependent upon an asynchronous development of stroke volume and arterial-venous oxygen difference. The stroke volume contributes most to the changes in $\dot{V}O_2$ throughout the growth phase, while $a - \bar{v}O_2$ difference shows a weaker relation in this period of development (24).

Presently there are no other longitudinal studies which have attempted to analyze the relative contributions of the heart and peripheral functional capacity to the development of the overall gas transport capacity. The exception to this appears to be the study of eight long-distance runners in Sweden (46). The boys were measured biannually from ages 12 to 15 and, during these tests, muscle fiber types and muscle cross-sectional area by tomography were measured in the vastus lateralis. The chronic endurance training during this period of growth did not alter the muscle fiber type. Changes in cross-sectional area correlated with strength development (peak torque). Longitudinal improvements in 1,000-meter running times were tightly coupled to the improved leg strength.

SUMMARY

The problems of studying how an organ system functions during growth have been described. Multiple confounding factors operating at different times make it impossible to interpret cross-sectional data or longitudinal data that is not normalized for growth and maturation patterns. An emphasis has been placed on those longitudinal studies that have recognized the importance of accounting for growth, maturation, and physical activity patterns when studying the changes in the cardiorespiratory system of children.

The association of body size with the development of the cardiorespiratory system appears to be fortuitous. Both size and function may be independent factors related to a common control — genetic endowment. Although the development of size and function appear to be independent during the growth years, the size ultimately predicts the capacity of the cardiorespiratory system. Body height has been used as the reference factor to describe the changes in this system among children.

Physical activity apparently modifies the size-to-capacity relationship. The influence of activity upon this system appears to be greatest when applied during the year preceding PHV and afterward; however, the concept of a critical age during which physical activity will modify the development of this system is speculative. Any exercise programs which have demonstrated changes in cardiorespiratory function are by nature very vigorous. They must add substantial intense periods of activity to a population group that is already spontaneously active.

Further data from completed longitudinal studies or additional information from suggested designs using twins or random allocation to group activity may add substantially to our understanding of the growth of this system. In particular, the use of noninvasive measures of physiological function to observe mechanisms of adaptation in children in response to growth, maturation, or activity may provide the necessary data for the detailed analyses of functional changes in the cardiorespiratory system.

REFERENCES

1. Akima, H. A new method of interpolation and smooth curve fitting based on local procedures. *J. Assoc. Comp. Mach.,* 17:589-602. 1970.

2. Anderson, K.L., J. Rutenfranz, and V. Seliger. The rate of growth in maximal aerobic power of children in Norway. *Medicine Sport,* 11:52-55, 1978.

3. Andrew, G.M., M.R. Becklace, J.S. Guleria, and D.V. Bates. Heart and lung functions in swimmers and non-athletes during growth. *J. Appl. Physiol.,* 32(2):245-251, 1972.

4. Asmussen, E., and K.R. Heeboll-Nielsen. A dimensional analysis of physical performance and growth in boys. *J. Appl. Physiol.,* 7:593-603, 1955.

5. Åstrand, P.-O., L. Engstrom, B.O. Eriksson, P. Karlberg, I. Nylander, B. Saltin, and C. Thoren. Girl swimmers. *Acta Paediatr.* (suppl. 147), 1963.

6. Åstrand, P.-O., K. Rodahl. *Textbook of work physiology,* p. 681. New York: McGraw-Hill, 1977.

7. Bailey, D.A. Exercise, fitness, and physical education for the growing child — A concern. *Can. J. Public Health,* 64:421-430, 1973.

8. Bailey, D.A., R.M. Malina, and R.L. Rasmussen. "The influence of exercise, physical activity, and athletic performance on the dynamics of human growth." In *Human growth, Vol. 2, Postnatal growth,* edited by F. Falkner and J.M. Tanner, pp. 475-505. New York: Plenum Press, 1978.

9. Bailey, D.A., W.D. Ross, R.L. Mirwald, and C. Weese. Size dissociation of maximal aerobic power during growth in boys. *Medicine Sport,* 11:140-151, 1978.

10. Bar-Or, O., R.J. Shephard, and C.L. Allen. Cardiac output of 10-to 13-year old boys and girls during submaximal exercise. *J. Appl. Physiol.,* 30(2):19-223, 1971.

11. Bar-Or, O., and L.D. Zwiren. "Physiological effects of increased frequency of physical education classes and of endurance conditioning on 9- to 10-year-old girls and boys." In *Pediatric work physiology, proceedings 4th international symposium,* pp. 183-198. Wingate Institute, Israel, 1973.

12. Berg, K., and J. Bjure. Preliminary results of long-term physical training of adolescent boys with respect to body composition, maximal oxygen uptake, and lung volume. *Acta Paediatr. Belg.,* 28:183-189, 1974.

13. Beunen, G., M. Ostyn, R. Benson, J. Simmons, P. Swalus, and D. Van Gerven. "Somatotype and physical fitness of 14-year-old boys." In *Frontiers of activity and child health,* edited by H. Lavallee and R.J. Shephard, pp. 115-123. Ottawa: Pelican, 1977.

14. Blimkie, C.J.R. *Gas transport capacity and cardiorespiratory function in 9- to 15-year-old boys during exercise in relation to growth, maturation, heart size and regular physical activity.* Unpublished thesis, University of Western Ontario, 1982.

15. Blimkie, C.J.R., D.A. Cunningham, and P.M. Nichol. Gas transport capacity and echocardiographically determined cardiac size in children. *J. Appl. Physiol.,* 49(6):994-999, 1980.

16. Boileau, R.A., A. Bonen, V.H. Heyward, and B.H. Massey. Maximal aerobic capacity on the treadmill and bicycle ergometer of boys 11-14 years of age *J. Sports Med.,* 7:153-162, 1977.

17. Bouchard, C. "Genetics, growth and physical activity." In *Physical activity and human well-being,* edited by F. Landry and W.A.R. Orban, pp. 29-45. Miami: Symposia Specialists, 1978.

18. Bouchard, C., R.M. Malina, W. Hollmann, and C. Leblanc. Submaximal working capacity, heart size and body size in boys 8-18 years. *Europ. J. Appl. Physiol.,* 36:115-126, 1977.

19. Brown, C.H., J.R. Harrower, and M.F. Deeter. The effects of cross-country running on pre-adolescent girls. *Med. Sci. Sports,* 4:1-5, 1972.

20. Cameron, N., R.L. Mirwald, and D.A. Bailey. "Standards for the assessment of normal absolute maximal aerobic power." In *Kinanthropometry II, international series on sport sciences,* Vol. 9, edited by M. Ostyn, G. Beunen, and J. Simons. Baltimore: University Park Press, 1980.

21. Cumming, G.R. Hemodynamics of supine bicycle exercise in "normal" children. *Amer. Heart J.,* 93:617-622, 1977.

22. Cunningham, D.A. "Physical working capacity of children and adolescents." In *Encyclopedia of physical education, fitness and sports,* edited by G.A. Stull and T.K. Cureton, Jr., pp. 481-494. Salt Lake City: Brighton Publ. Co., 1980.

23. Cunningham, D.A., and R.B. Eynon. The working capacity of young competitive swimmers, 10-16 years of age. *Med. Sci. Sports,* 5:227-231, 1973.

24. Cunningham, D.A., D.H. Paterson, C.J.R. Blimkie, and A.P. Donner. Development of cardiorespiratory function in circumpubertal boys: A longitudinal study. *J. Appl. Physiol.: Respirat. Environ. Exer. Physiol.,* 56(2):302-307, 1984.

25. Cunningham, D.A., J.J. Stapleton, I.C. MacDonald, and D.H. Paterson. Daily energy expenditure of young boys as related to maximal aerobic power. *Can. J. Appl. Spt. Sci.,* 6:207-211, 1981.

26. Cunningham, D.A., P. Telford, and G.T. Swart. The cardiopulmonary capacities of young hockey players: Age 10. *Med. Sci. Sports,* 8:23-25, 1976.

27. Cunningham, D.A., B. Van Waterschoot, D.H. Paterson, M.

Lefcoe, and S.P. Sangal. Reliability and reproducibility of maximal oxygen uptake measurements in children. *Med. Sci. Sports*, 9(2):104-108, 1977.

28. Daniels, J., and N. Oldridge. Changes in oxygen consumption of young boys during growth and running training. *Med. Sci. Sports*, 3:161-165, 1971.

29. Davies, C.T.M., C. Barnes, and S. Godfrey. Body composition and maximal exercise performance in children. *Hum. Biol.*, 44(3): 195-214, 1972.

30. Ekblom, B. Effect of physical training in adolescent boys. *J. Appl. Physiol.*, 27(3):350-355, 1969.

31. Eriksson, B.O., P.D. Gollnick, and B. Saltin. The effect of physical training on muscle enzyme activities and fiber composition in 11-year-old boys. *Acta Paediat. Belgica*, 28 (Suppl.):245-252, 1974.

32. Eriksson, B.O., G. Grimby, and B. Saltin. Cardiac output and arterial blood gases during exercise in pubertal boys. *J. Appl. Physiol.*, 31(3):348-352, 1971.

33. Eriksson, B.O., and G. Koch. Effect of physical training on hemodynamic response during submaximal and maximal exercise in 11-to 13-year-old boys. *Acta Physiol. Scand.*, 87:27-39, 1973.

34. Fahey, T.D., A. Del Valle-Zuris, G. Oehlsen, M. Trieb, and J. Seymour. Pubertal stage differences in hormonal and hematological responses to maximal exercise in males. *J. Appl. Physiol.: Respirat. Environ. Exercise Physiol.*, 46:823-827, 1979.

35. Gadhoke, S., and N.L. Jones. The responses to exercise in boys aged 9-15 years. *Clin. Sci.*, 37:789-801, 1969.

36. Gilliam, T.B., P.S. Freedson, D.L. Greenen, and B. Shahrary. Physical activity patterns determined by heart rate monitoring in 6-to 7-year-old children. *Med. Sci. Sports Exercise*, 13:65-67, 1981.

37. Gilliam, T.B., S. Sady, W.G. Thorland, and A.L. Weltman. Comparison of peak performance measures in children ages 6 to 8, 9 to 10, and 11 to 13 years. *Res. Quart.*, 48(4):695-702, 1977.

38. Godfrey, S. "The growth and development of the cardiopulmonary responses to exercise." In *Scientific foundations of paediatrics*, edited by J. Dobbing and J.A. Davis, pp. 271-280. Philadelphia: Saunders, 1974.

39. Godfrey, S. *Exercise testing in children*, p. 168. London, Saunders, 1974.

40. Godfrey, S., C.T.M. Davies, E. Wozniak, and C.A. Barnes. Cardiorespiratory response to exercise in normal children. *Clin. Sci.*, 40:419-431, 1971.

41. Goode, R.C., A. Virgin, T.T. Romet, P. Crawford, J. Duffin, T. Pallandi, and Z. Woch. Effects of a short period of physical activity in adolescent boys and girls. *Can. J. Appl. Spt. Sci.*, 1:241-250, 1976.

42. Hamilton, P., and G.M. Andrew. Influence of growth and athletic training on heart and lung functions. *Europ. J. Appl. Physiol.,* 36:27-28, 1976 .

43. Hermansen, L., and S. Oseid. Direct and indirect estimation of maximal oxygen uptake in pre-pubertal boys. *Acta Paediatr. Scand.* (suppl. 217):18-23, 1971.

44. Hockey, R.V., and M.C. Howe. "Changes occurring in cardiovascular endurance during a season of competitive hockey for 13- and 14-year-old boys and relation of selected tests to maximal $\dot{V}O_2$." In *Science in skiing, skating and hockey,* edited by J. Terauds and H.J. Gros, pp. 139-150. Del Mar: Academic Publishers, 1979.

45. Howald, H. Ultrastructure and biochemical function of skeletal muscle in twins. *Ann. Hum. Biol.,* 3:80 (Abstract), 1976.

46. Jacobs, I., B. Sjodin, and B. Svaue. Muscle fiber type, cross-sectional area and strength in boys after 4 years endurance training. *Med. Sci. Sports Exer.,* 14:123 (Abstract), 1982.

47. Kellet, D.W., P.L.T. Willan, and K.J. Bagnall. A study of potential Olympic swimmers. Part 2. Changes due to three months intensive training. *Brit. J. Sports Med.,* 12(2):87-92, 1978.

48. Kemper, H.C.G., and R. Verschuur. Validity and reliability of pedometers in research on habitual physical activity. In *Frontiers of activity and child health,* edited by H. Lavallee and R.J. Shephard, pp. 83-92. Ottawa: Editions du Pelican, 1977.

49. Kemper, H.C.G., and R. Verschuur. Maximal aerobic power in 13- and 14-year-old teenagers in relation to biologic age. *Int. J. Sports Med.,* 2:97-100, 1981.

50. Kemper, H.C.G., R. Verschuur, K.G.A. Ras, J. Snel, P.G. Splinter, and L.W.E. Tavecchio. Investigation into the effects of two extra physical education lessons per week during one school year upon the physical development of 12- and 13-year-old boys. *Medicine Sport,* 11:159-166, 1978.

51. Kleiber, M. Body size conductance for animal heat flow in Newton's Law of cooling. *J. Thear. Biol.,* 37:139-150, 1972.

52. Klissouras, V. Heritability of adaptive variation. *J. Appl. Physiol.,* 31:338-344, 1971.

53. Klissouras, V. "Genetic aspects of physical fitness." In *Physical fitness,* edited by V. Seliger, pp. 217-223. Praugue: Universita Karlova, 1973.

54. Kobayashi, K., K. Kitamura, M. Miura, H. Sodeyama, Y. Murase, M. Miyashita, and H. Matsui. Aerobic power as related to body growth and training in Japanese boys: A longitudinal study. *J. Appl. Physiol.: Respirat. Environ. Exercise Physiol.,* 44(5):666-672, 1978.

55. Koch, G. Aerobic power, lung dimensions, ventilatory capacity, and muscle blood flow in 12- 16-year-old boys with high physical activi-

ty. In *Children and exercise* IX, edited by K. Berg and B. Eriksson, pp. 99-108. Baltimore: University Park Press, 1980.

56. Koch, G., and B.O. Eriksson. Effect of physical training on pulmonary ventilation and gas exchange during submaximal and maximal work in boys aged 11 to 13 years. *Scand. J. Clin. Lab. Invest.*, 31:87-94, 1973.

57. Komi, P.V., and J. Karlsson. Physical performance, skeletal muscle enzyme activities, and fiber types in monozygous and dizygous twins of both sexes. *Acta Physiol. Scand.* (Suppl. 462), 1979.

58. Komi, P.V., J.H.T. Viitasalo, M. Havu, A. Thorstensson, B. Sjodin, and J. Karlsson. Skeletal muscle fibres and muscle enzyme activities in monozygous and dizygous twins of both sexes. *Acta Physiol. Scand.*, 100:385, 1977.

59. Leitch, A.G. Chemical control of breathing in identical twin athletes. *Ann. Human Biol.*, 3:447 (Abstract), 1976.

60. Lussier, L., and E.R. Buskirk. Effect of an endurance training regimen on assessment of work capacity in prepubertal children. *Ann. N.Y. Acad. Sci.*, 301:734-747, 1977.

61. Malina, R.M. "Physical activity, growth, and functional capacity." In *Human physical growth and maturation. Methodologies and factors*, edited by F.E. Johnson, A.F. Roche, and C. Susanne, pp. 161-175. New York: Plenum Press, 1980.

62. Marshall, W.A. "*Puberty*". In *Human growth, Vol. 2, Postnatal growth*, edited by F. Falkner and J.M. Tanner, pp. 141-181. New York: Plenum Press, 1978.

63. Massicotte, D.R., and R.B.J. MacNab. Cardiorespiratory adaptations to training at specified intensities in children. *Med. Sci. Sports*, 66:242-246, 1974.

64. McMiken, D.F. Maximum aerobic power and physical dimensions of children. *Ann. Human Biol.*, 3:141-147, 1976.

65. Mirwald, R.L. "Saskatchewan growth and development study." In *Kinanthropometry II, international series on sport sciences* (Vol. 9), pp. 289-305. Baltimore: University Park Press, 1980.

66. Mirwald, R.L., D.A. Bailey, N. Cameron, and R.L. Rasmussen. Longitudinal comparison of aerobic power in active and inactive boys aged 7.0 to 17.0 years. *Ann. Human Biol.*, 8(5):405-414, 1981.

67. Miyamura, M., and Y. Honda. Maximum cardiac output related to sex and age. *Jap. J. Physiol.*, 23:645-656, 1973.

68. Mocellin. R., and U. Wasmund. "Investigations on the influence of a running-training program on the cardiovascular and motor performance capacity in 53 boys and girls of a second and third primary school class." In *Pediatric work physiology, proceedings of 4th international symposium*, pp. 279-285. Wingate Institute, Israel, 1973.

69. Paterson, D.H., and D.A. Cunningham. Comparison of methods

to calculate cardiac output using the CO_2 rebreathing method. *Europ. J. Appl. Physiol.*, 35:223-230, 1976.

70. Paterson, D.H., D.A. Cunningham, and A. Donner. The effect of different treadmill speeds on the variability of $\dot{V}O_2$max in children. *Eur. J. Appl. Physiol.*, 47:113-122, 1981.

71. Paterson, D.H., D.A. Cunningham, D.S. Penny, M. Lefcoe, and S. Sangal. Heart rate telemetry and estimated energy metabolism in minor league ice hockey. *Can. J. Appl. Spt. Sci.*, 2:71-75, 1977.

72. Paterson, D.H., D.A. Cunningham, M.J. Plyley, C.J.R. Blimkie, and A.P. Donner. The consistency of cardiac output measurement (CO_2 rebreathe) in children during exercise. *Eur. J. Appl. Physiol.*, 49:37-44, 1982.

73. Preece, M.A., and M.J. Baines. A new family of mathematical models describing the human growth curve. *Ann. Human Biol.*, 5:1-24, 1978.

74. Renson, R., G. Beunen, M. Ostyn, J. Simons, and D. van Gerven. Family constellation and physical fitness of 12- to 19-year-old Belgian boys. *International Symposium, growth and development of the child* (Abstract), Trois-Rivières, P.Q., 1980

75. Ross, W.D., D.A. Bailey, and C.H. Weese. "Proportionality in interpretation of longitudinal metabolic function data on boys." In *Frontiers of activity and child health*, edited by H. Lavallee and R.J. Shephard, pp. 225-236. Ottawa: Editions du Pelican, 1977.

76. Rutenfranz, J., K.L. Anderson, V. Seliger, F. Klimmer, I. Berndt, and M. Ruppel. Maximum aerobic power and body composition during the puberty growth period: Similarities and differences between children of two European countries. *Eur. J. Pediatr.*, 136:123-133, 1981.

77. Schumacker, B., and W. Hollman. The aerobic capacity of trained athletes from 6 to 7 years of age. *Acta Paediatr. Belgica*, 28 (suppl.):91-101, 1974.

78. Seely, J.E., C.A. Guzman, and M.R. Becklace. Heart and lung function at rest and during exercise in adolescents. *J. Appl. Physiol.*, 36(1):34-40, 1974.

79. Seliger, V. The influence of sports training on the efficiency of juniors. *Int. Z. Angew. Physiol.*, 26:309-322, 1968.

80. Shasby, G.B., and F.C. Hagerman. The effects of conditioning on cardiorespiratory function in adolescent boys. *J. Sports Med.* May/June:97-107, 1975.

81. Shephard, R.J. *Human physiological work capacity*, pp. 301-303. Cambridge: Cambridge University Press, 1978.

82. Shephard, R.J., H. Lavallee, M. Rijic, J-C. Jequier, C. Beaucage, and R. LaGarre. "Influence of added activity classes upon the working capacity of Quebec school children." In *Frontiers of activity and child health*, edited by H. Lavallee and R.J. Shephard, pp. 237-245. Ottawa: Editions du Pelican, 1977.

83. Sjodin, B. Lactate dehydrogenase in human skeletal muscle. *Acta Physiol. Scand.* (Suppl. 436), 1976.

84. Skinner, J.S., O. Bar-Or, V. Bergsteinova, C.W. Bell, D. Roger, and E.R. Buskirk. Comparison of continuous and intermittent tests for determining maximal oxygen intake in children. *Acta Paediatr. Scand.* (Suppl.) 217:24-28, 1971.

85. Sprynarova, S. Development of the relationship between aerobic capacity and the circulatory and respiratory reaction to moderate activity in boys 11-13 years old. *Physiol. Bohemoslov.*, 15(3):253-264, 1966.

86. Sprynarova, S. Longitudinal study of the influence of different physical activity programs on functional capacity of the boys from 11 to 18 years. *Acta Paediatr. Belgica*, 28:204-213, 1974.

87. Sprynarova, S., J. Pařizkova, and I. Jurmora. Development of the functional capacity and body composition of boy and girl swimmers aged 12-15 years. *Medicine Sport*, 11:32-38, 1978.

88. Stewart, K.J., and B. Gutin. The prediction of maximal oxygen uptake before and after physical training in children. *J. Human Ergol.*, 4:153-162, 1975.

89. Stewart, K.J., and B. Gutin. Effects of physical training on cardiorespiratory fitness in children. *Res. Quart. Amer. Assoc. Health Phys. Educ.*, 47:110-120, 1976.

90. Stoboy, H. "Stroke volume and cardiac output in ergometric performance." In *Ergometry, basics of medical exercise testing*, edited by H. Mellerowicz and V.N. Smodlaka, pp. 89-121. Baltimore: Urban and Schwarzenberg. (Translated by A.L. Rice), 1981.

91. Tanner, J.M. "Growth and endocrinology of the adolescent." In *Endocrine and genetic diseases of childhood and adolescence*, edited by L.I. Gardner, pp. 14-64. Philadelphia: Saunders, 1975.

92. Tanner, J.M., R.H. Whitehouse, and M. Takaishi. Standards from birth to maturity for height, weight velocity: British children, 1965. *Arch. Dis. of Childh.*, 41:454-471, 1966.

93. Thomas, S.G., D.A. Cunningham, M.J. Plyley, D.R. Boughen, and R.A. Cook. Central and peripheral adaptations of the gas transport system to one-leg training *Can. J. Physiol. Pharmacol.*, 59:1146-1154, 1981.

94. Thomson, M.J., D.A. Cunningham, and G.A. Wearring. Eating habits and caloric intake of physically active young boys, aged 10 to 14 years. *Can. J. Appl. Spt. Sci.*, 5:10-14, 1980.

95. Vanfraechem, J.H.P., and R. Vanfraechem-Raway. The influence of training upon physiological and psychological parameters in young athletes. *J. Sports Med.*, 18:175-182, 1978.

96. Von Dobeln, W., and B.O. Eriksson. Physical training, maximal oxygen uptake and dimensions of the oxygen transporting and metabolizing organs in boys 11-13 years of age. *Acta Paediatr. Scand.*, 61:653-660, 1972.

97. Weber, G., W. Kartodihardjo, and V. Klissouras. Growth and physical training with reference to heredity. *J. Appl. Physiol.,* 40(2):211-215, 1976.

98. Wells, C.L., E.W. Scrutton, L.D. Archibald, W.P. Cooke, and J.W. De La Mothe. Physical working capacity and maximal oxygen uptake of teenaged athletes. *Med. Sci. Sports.,* 5(4):232-238, 1973.

99. Wolfe, L.A., and D.A. Cunningham. Effects of chronic exercise on cardiac output and its determinants. *Can. J. Physiol. Pharmacol.,* 60:1089-1097, 1982.

100. Yamaji, K., and M. Miyashita. Oxygen transport system during exhaustive exercise in Japanese boys. *Europ. J. Appl. Physiol.,* 36:93-99, 1977.

5

Children and Physical Performance in Warm and Cold Environments

Oded Bar-Or

McMaster University and Chedoke-McMaster Hospitals

When heat or cold is superimposed on the stress of physical exercise, the performance and well-being of the child may be compromised. This chapter will review the responses of children and adolescents to these combined stresses. Rather than systematically analyzing thermoregulation during exercise, the review will emphasize *differences* in the thermoregulatory responses of children, adolescents, and adults. For basic concepts of environmental physiology, the reader should consult previous reviews (11,21) or textbooks of environmental physiology (33,41).

Even though epidemiologic studies have long suggested that infants and children do not fare well in hot climates (18,43), systematic research on the thermoregulation of the exercising child is a young field of investigation. One reason for the paucity of data in this area is the ethical considerations. Protocols for studying responses to heat or cold call for exposing the individual to "hostile" environments or inducing shifts in body water compartments, procedures that are hard to justify with children. Furthermore, invasive techniques, often performed with adult volunteers, cannot readily be used with children.

There are also methodological constraints in comparing thermoregulation among different age groups. For example, how should metabolic loads be equated among subjects? (Results could be expressed per kg body weight, as percent of maximal aerobic power, or as percent of maximal heart rate.) What weight should be assigned to different skin sites to determine mean skin temperature? What proportions should be used for body core and periphery in the calculation of mean body temperature? Should the same "end points" used with adults to terminate an exposure to work in the heat or work in the cold be used with children? As a result of such ethical and methodological constraints, our knowledge of age- or maturation-related differences in thermoregulation is based on a fragmentary body of data and is still somewhat speculative.

This chapter will first review the physiologic aspects of children's exercise in hot and cold environments, followed by implications for performance and health of the sick and the healthy child. Finally, ideas for further research in this challenging field will be suggested.

THERMOREGULATORY CONSTRAINTS
AND THE EXERCISING CHILD

A number of morphologic and functional characteristics of children make them less efficient thermoregulators than adults. These include:

1. large surface area per body mass unit,

2. high oxygen cost of walking and running,

3. lower cardiac output at a given oxygen uptake, and

4. lower sweating rate.

The relatively large body surface area is conducive to greater heat exchange between the skin and the environment, namely, heat gain when ambient temperature exceeds skin temperature and heat loss when the body is exposed to the cold. Excessive heat gain in warm climates, which is particularly pronounced at high air-to-skin temperature gradients, is a definite liability during exercise. The greater heat loss is beneficial when ambient temperature is somewhat lower than skin temperature (e.g., air temperature of 20-22°C), but it becomes a liability in cooler weather and especially when the child is immersed in water.

The high oxygen cost of locomotion has been described for children (4) and confirmed in various studies (13,34,44). The implication for thermoregulation is that children at a given speed of walking or running produce more metabolic heat per kilogram body weight than do adolescents or adults. This presents a greater strain on the heat dissipating systems of the young.

Cardiac output at a given metabolic level is somewhat lower, and stroke volume is markedly lower, in children than it is in older persons (10,17,19). This presents a potential handicap during intense exercise in the heat, when the demand for increased blood flow to the myocardium, skeletal muscles, lungs, and skin may not be met. Insufficient blood supply to the skin may interfere with the convection of heat from the body core to the periphery, while insufficient perfusion of the lungs and muscles may impede oxygen transport during intense exercise.

Another age-related hemodynamic difference has been shown between prepubertal girls and young women who exercise in the heat (17). The girls responded with a shift of central blood volume to the periphery, which could explain the reduction in stroke volume due to the decrease in venous return. Such a shift was not apparent among adult women.

Perhaps the major difference in thermoregulation between children and older age groups is in the sweating pattern, as summarized in Table 5-1. The sweating rate of prepubertal children is distinctly lower than that of older age groups, whether defined in absolute volume or per unit surface area. Whereas postpubertal adolescents or adults can perspire at rates exceeding 500-600 ml per square meter of skin per hour during moderate exercise in the heat, the child's perspiration seldom exceeds 350 ml per square meter per hour while exposed to identical conditions (3,17,27). A similar difference exists when exercise is performed in a neutral climate (14). Figure 5-1 shows the difference in the sweating rate of prepubertal and pubertal boys. It has been claimed (46), but not confirmed, that the sweating rate is related to the level of circulating androgens during puberty.

The lower sweating rate in children is due to a lower output of each sweat gland rather than to a smaller population density of heat-activated sweat glands (6). This low output per gland is also evident during pilocarpine iontophoresis (26), suggesting that a reduced local response rather than lower sympathetic drive is responsible for the child's sweating pattern. Another possible cause for a low sweat production is the smaller cross-sectional area of the gland's acinus in children (32).

Table 5-1

Sweating Patterns During Exercise—Comparisons Between Prepubertal Children and Young Adults

Variable	Response of Children (Compared With Adults)	References
Sweating rate— absolute values	Lower	Araki et al. (3) Davies (14) Drinkwater et al. (17) Inbar (27)
Sweating rate— per unit surface area	Lower	Ibid
Sweat output per gland	2.5 times lower	Bar-Or (6)
Population density of heat-activated sweat glands	Lower	Bar-Or (6)
Chloride concentration in sweat	Lower	Araki et al. (3) Dill et al. (16)
Set point (Δ rectal temp. at which sweating starts)	Higher	Araki et al. (3)
Conditioning-induced increase in sweating rate	Attenuated	Araki (2) Araki et al. (3)

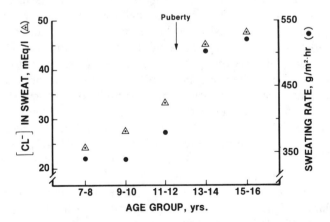

Figure 5-1. Age-related changes in sweating rate and in chloride concentration in the sweat. Subjects were 40 Japanese boys, 7 to 16 years old, exercising on a cycle ergometer at heart rates of 160-170 beat/min. Sweating rate was determined from changes in body weight. Sweat for chloride analysis was collected from the pectoralis major area. Based on data by Araki et al. (3).

TOLERANCE TO EXERCISE
IN WARM AND COLD ENVIRONMENTS

The ability to complete a predetermined physical task or to sustain optimal exercise performance in hostile climates is often referred to as
tolerance. Table 5-2 is a summary comparing the tolerance of children
and adults to exercise in various environments.

The highest climatic heat stress in which children can sustain exercise is
lower than that for adults (17,24 vs. 9,48). For example, when given a
60-minute walking task at 4.8 km/hr, 0-5% grade, girls (9-11 years) and
women (19-22 years) completed all walks at climatic conditions equal to
or cooler than 29.4°C effective temperature (43°C, 13% relative humidity). However, when exposed to 32.2°C effective temperature (50°C, 13%
relative humidity) the girls had to stop their walk after 43 minutes while
the women managed to complete the prescribed task (24 vs. 9). The in-
ability of these girls and those in other studies to complete the walk was
apparent, even though their rectal temperature at the stage of termination was seldom higher than 38.5°C (6,17). It has been suggested,
although yet to be confirmed, that cardiovascular strain rather than thermoregulatory insufficiency caused the girls to terminate their walk (17).

Another criterion for exercise tolerance in warm environments is the
"prescriptive zone," that is, the range of ambient conditions in which
body core temperature remains unchanged at a given metabolic level,
regardless of the environmental stress. This range is the same for

Table 5-2

Tolerance of Children to Prolonged Exercise in Warm, Neutral, and Cool Environments—Comparison With Young Adults

Variable	Response of Children (Compared With Adults)	References
Highest climatic heat stress tolerated	Lower	Drinkwater et al. (17) Haymes et al. (24) vs. Bar-Or et al. (9)
Prescriptive zone	Same	Bar-Or (6)
Tolerance in neutral climate	Same/somewhat lower	Davies (14) Gullestad (23)
Tolerance in cool water	Lower	Sloan & Keatinge (45)
Tolerance in cold air	No data	

prepubertal children and adults of both sexes (6,25,39) and suggests that at mild and moderate heat stresses, exercising children are *not* at a handicap, at least not for moderately strenuous tasks (e.g., 40-50% of their maximal aerobic power).

In neutral climates children's exercise tolerance seems to be the same as that of adults, as is their thermoregulatory capacity (14,23,35,37). This is seen in spite of a lesser use by children of evaporative cooling and a greater reliance on heat dissipation through convection and radiation (14).

In cool climates, children seem to fare well when exercising on land, at least at intensities that produce sufficient metabolic heat to offset heat loss. However, there are no studies that systematically assess their thermoregulatory capability under these conditions. In contrast, when children exercise in water they lose greater amounts of heat and their core temperature drops faster than that of adolescents and young adults (45). The reason for such excessive cooling is that water has a markedly greater thermal conductivity than does air, thus enhancing heat loss by conduction from the skin. Such heat loss is exaggerated in children due to their large surface area.

Figure 5-2 is an attempt to compare the thermoregulatory ability of children and adults. When exercising in air temperature that is lower than skin temperature by some 5 to 15°C, children thermoregulate as effectively as adults. However, when air temperature approaches skin temperature the child cannot benefit from his/her greater convective or radiative potential and must resort to sweating as the only heat dissipating mechanism. At this stage his/her ability to dissipate heat is

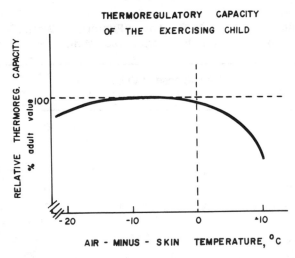

Figure 5-2. A schematic presentation of the relationship between thermoregulatory capacity and the air-to-skin temperature gradient. The capacity of children is plotted as percentage of that of adults, taking adult values as 100%.

deficient compared with the adult. At higher environmental temperatures the child's greater surface area becomes a handicap. The greater the air-to-skin temperature gradient, the less effective is the child as a thermoregulator. One can assume that a similar pattern evolves when air temperature is considerably *lower* than skin temperature.

ACCLIMATIZATION TO EXERCISE IN THE HEAT

Children, like adults, acclimatize to exercise in the heat by a reduction in heart rate, core and skin temperatures, and by an increase in sweating rate and in the sensitivity of the sweating apparatus to a rise in core temperature.

While the overall acclimatization attained by children is not dissimilar to that of adults (29,48) there are some age- or maturation-related differences in the pattern of acclimatization. These are summarized in Table 5-3.

When exposed to five sessions of cycling at dry heat (43°C dry bulb and 24°C wet bulb), 8- to 10-year-old boys had a distinctly slower rate of acclimatization than observed for 20- to 23-year-old men of similar maximal aerobic power (29). While physiologic changes compatible with partial acclimatization were seen in adults as early as the second session, it was not until the fourth session that similar changes were seen in children. The cause of such a slow rate of acclimatization in children is not known.

In order to acclimatize to exercise in the heat, adults require exposure to the combined stresses of heat and exercise; boys, however, can ac-

Table 5-3

Acclimatization of Children to Exercise In the Heat—
Comparison With Young Adults

Variable	Response of Children (Compared With Adults)	References
Ability to acclimatize	Adequate	Inbar et al. (29) Wagner et al. (48)
Speed of acclimatization	Slower	Bar-Or (6)
Acclimatization by conditioning in neutral climate	Better	Inbar et al. (28)
Acclimatization by resting in the heat	Better	Inbar et al. (30)

climatize also while resting passively in dry heat (30). Again, it is unclear why such a difference exists between the age groups. One possibility is that, due to their relatively large surface area, children are exposed to a greater effective heat stress at high ambient temperatures and this subjects their thermoregulatory apparatus to a higher strain relative to the adults even while at rest. It has yet to be determined whether passive exposures to warm, humid climates, in which ambient temperature does not exceed skin temperature, can also yield acclimatization in children.

In adults, conditioned individuals acclimatize more effectively than unconditioned individuals. There is still a controversy, however, as to whether conditioning in a neutral climate can induce acclimatization to heat (22). In 8- to 10-year-old boys, conditioning *per se* (exercise at 85% maximal heart rate) in 23°C, 50% relative humidity elicited the same level of acclimatization as was achieved through combined exercise and dry heat (28). It is possible that the children who exercise in neutral climates acclimatize primarily through cardiovascular changes (facilitating better convection from body core to periphery), whereas those who are exposed to exercise in the heat improve both their cardiovascular function and their evaporative capacity. Further knowledge of the acclimatization pattern of children is relevant not only to the physiologist but also to the health practitioner, since lack of acclimatization is a major cause of heat-related diseases.

FLUID AND ELECTROLYTE CHANGES DURING EXERCISE IN THE HEAT

Scant data are available to compare the fluid and electrolyte balance of children and adults who exercise in the heat. Adults who exercise intensely for a few minutes have a biphasic reduction in plasma volume. During the first few seconds fluid escapes the intravascular space due to an increase in intracapillary hydrostatic pressure. This is followed by a further reduction in plasma volume, probably due to a transcapillary osmotic differential secondary to efflux of potassium ions and metabolites from the contracting muscle. During supramaximal activity, a reduction in plasma volume of 10-15% is discerned within 30 seconds, as shown for young adults (40) and for children (Rotstein & Bar-Or, unpublished data).

During prolonged activities (30 minutes or more) total body water and plasma volume are further reduced whenever fluid intake does not fully replenish fluid loss. The latter is especially evident in warm climates where perspiration is marked. It has been suggested that during a 1-hour exercise in a neutral climate, the child's reduction in plasma volume is less than that found for adults. Moreover, when intensity of such prolonged exercise is low (40% of maximal aerobic power) children have a mild *increase* in plasma volume (36). However, these observations need further confirmation.

No studies are available in which fluid restriction was enforced upon exercising children. It has been shown that prepubertal boys, however, when exposed to intermittent exercise in dry heat (45% maximal aerobic power, 39°C, 45% relative humidity), dehydrate voluntarily even when allowed to drink *ad libitum* (8). The rate of dehydration under such conditions is not dissimilar to that described for adults. It seems, however, that the children had a greater rise in core temperature than did young adults at an equal percentage of body fluid deficit.

Knowledge of the extent and mechanisms of body fluid shifts is needed to further understand the thermoregulation of the exercising child. Such knowledge is also relevant to the health and well-being of the young athlete, especially in sports in which "making weight" by dehydration is commonly practiced. Observations among high school wrestlers have shown that some, especially in the lower weight categories, lose as much as 15% of initial body weight during the 10 days prior to a match (47). Assuming that most of such weight loss reflects hypohydration, it is highly likely that such children risk heat-related illness and possibly other diseases.

Studies that conform to proper epidemiologic principles are needed to define the actual hypohydration-induced risk to health. For ethical reasons, such studies may not be launched. However, anecdotal data do suggest that marked hypohydration (i.e., more than 10%) involves a definite risk to the health of young athletes (12).

As shown in Figure 5-1 and documented in various studies (3,16), children's sweat has lower salt concentration than that of adults. Values seldom reach 40 mEq/l in prepubertal boys while they often exceed to 60 mEq/l in more mature individuals. No data are available on the possible mechanisms or implications of such a difference. Nor is it known whether other ionic changes, described for the exercising adult, are also found in children.

IMPLICATIONS FOR HEALTH

Does the relatively deficient thermoregulatory capacity of children connote an increased risk to health? Retrospective observations suggest that during climatic heat waves, infants and children are more prone to heat-related illness than are young adults (18,43). However, there are no studies which define the actual incidence of heat-related illness in child athletes. With the advent of "fun runs" and other such races it may become possible to construct such studies.

Various groups of children, adolescents, and adults are at special risk of suffering heat-related illness during exercise in warm climates. These include healthy individuals who are hypohydrated or insufficiently acclimatized (5,20) and persons with a low fitness level, as well as patients with anorexia nervosa (15), congenital heart disease (38), cystic fibrosis (31), diabetes insipidus, diabetes mellitus, diarrhea, fever, malnutrition, obesity (25), prior heat illness (42), sweating insufficiency syndromes, and vomiting. The ability of these conditions to cause heat-related illness in children is reviewed elsewhere (6,7). The American Academy of Pediatrics (1) has published guidelines for children during athletic events in warm climates, and similar guidelines have been formulated in a text-book on pediatric sports medicine (7).

CHALLENGES FOR THE FUTURE

The age-related differences in response to exercise in warm and cold climates present an open field for further research. There are numerous unanswered theoretical questions on the maturation of the thermoregulatory capacity, as well as practical issues relating to health and performance. The following are some topics for further study, not chosen in order of priority but on the basis of the author's own bias.

- What are the *long-range sequelae* of repeated dehydration during growth? (e.g. stunted growth? renal calculi?)

- What *mechanisms* underlie the differences in acclimatization to heat between children and adults?

- Is the *sweating pattern* of children (many active glands secreting small volume of sweat) a handicap or an advantage (representing a more economical way for evaporative cooling)?

- What, if any, *hormonal* factors affect sweating and other thermoregulatory mechanisms during puberty?

- What are the *sex-related* differences in thermoregulation of prepubertal children?

- Are children prone to excessive heat loss when exercising on land in extremely cold environments (e.g., ice-skating or cross-country skiing)?

- Do girls acclimatize to exercise in the heat as effectively as boys?

In addition, studies based on sound epidemiologic principles are needed concerning the incidence and severity of heat-related illness among child athletes.

REFERENCES

1. American Academy of Pediatrics Committee On Sports Medicine. Climatic heat stress and the exercising child. *Pediatrics*, 69:808-809, 1982.

2. Araki, T. The effect of physical training on sweating responses measured during muscular exercises and resting postures in hot environments. *Kobe J. Med. Sci.,* 22:17-33, 1976.

3. Araki, T., Y. Toda, K. Matsushita, and A. Tsujino. Age differences in sweating during muscular exercise. *Jap. J. Phys. Fitness Sports Med.,* 28:239-248, 1979.

4. Åstrand, P.O., *Experimental studies of physical working capacity in relation to sex and age.* Copenhagen: Munksgaard, 1952.

5. Barcenas, C., H.P. Hoeffler, and J.T. Lie. Obesity, football, dog days and siriasis: A deadly combination. *Amer. Heart J.,* 92:237-244, 1976.

6. Bar-Or, O. Climate and the exercising child—A review. *Int. J. Sports Med.,* 1:53-65, 1980.

7. Bar-Or, O. *Pediatric sports medicine: From physiologic principles to clinical application.* New York: Springer Verlag, 1983.

8. Bar-Or, O., R. Dotan, O. Inbar, A. Rotshtein, and H. Zonder. Voluntary hypohydration in 10- to 12-year-old boys. *J. Appl. Physiol.: Respirat. Environ. Exercise Physiol.,* 48:104-108, 1980.

9. Bar-Or, O., H.M. Lundegren, and E.R. Buskirk. Heat tolerance of exercising obese and lean women. *J. Appl. Physiol.,* 26:403-409, 1969.

10. Bar-Or, O., R.J. Shephard, and C.L. Allen. Cardiac output of 10-to 13-year-old boys and girls during submaximal exercise. *J. Appl. Physiol.,* 30:219-223, 1971.

11. Brengelmann, G.L. Circulatory adjustments to exercise and heat stress. *Ann. Rev. Physiol.,* 45: 191-212, 1983.

12. Croyle, P.H., R.A. Place, and A.D. Hilgenberg. Massive pulmonary embolism in a high school wrestler. *JAMA,* 241:827-828, 1979.

13. Daniels, J., N. Oldridge, F. Nagle, and B. White. Differences and changes in $\dot{V}O_2$ among young runners 10 to 18 years of age. *Med. Sci. Sports,* 10:200-203, 1978.

14. Davies, C.T.M. Thermal responses to exercise in children. *Ergonomics,* 24:55-61, 1981.

15. Davies, C.T.M., L. Fohlin, and C. Thorén. "Thermoregulation in anorexia patients." In *Pediatric work physiology,* edited by J. Borms and M. Hebbelinck, pp. 96-101. Basel: Karger, 1978.

16. Dill, D.B., F.G. Hall, and W. Van Beaumont. Sweat chloride concentration: Sweat rate, metabolic rate, skin temperature, and age. *J. Appl. Physiol.,* 21:99-106, 1966.

17. Drinkwater, B.L., I.C. Kupprat, J.E. Denton, J.L. Crist, and S.M. Horvath. Response of prepubertal girls and college women to work in the heat. *J. Appl. Physiol.: Respirat. Environ. Exercise Physiol.,* 43:1046-1053, 1977.

18. Ellis, F.P., A.N. Exton Smith, K.G. Foster, and J.S. Weiner. Eccrine sweating and mortality during heat waves in very young and very old persons. *Israel J. Med. Sci.,* 12:815-817, 1976.

19. Eriksson, B.O. Cardiac output during exercise in pubertal boys. *Acta Paediatr. Scand.,* Suppl. 217:53-55, 1971.

20. Fox, E.L., D.K. Mathews, W.S. Kaufman, and R.W. Bowers. Effects of football equipment on thermal balance and energy cost during exercise. *Res. Quart. Amer. Assoc. Health Phys. Ed. Recr.,* 37:332-339, 1966.

21. Gisolfi, C.V. Temperature regulation during exercise: Directions — 1983. *Med. Sci. Sports Exerc.,* 15:15-20, 1983.

22. Gisolfi, C.V., and J.S. Cohen. Relationship among training, heat acclimatization and heat tolerance in men and women: The controversy revisited. *Med. Sci. Sports,* 11:56-59, 1979.

23. Gullestad, R. Temperature regulation in children during exercise. *Acta Paediatr. Scand.,* 64:257-263, 1975.

24. Haymes, E.M., E.R. Buskirk, J.L. Hodgson, H.M. Lundegren, and W.C. Nicholas. Heat tolerance of exercising lean and heavy prepubertal girls. *J. Appl. Physiol.,* 36:566-571, 1974.

25. Haymes, E.M., R.J. McCormick, and E.R. Buskirk. Heat tolerance of exercising lean and obese prepubertal boys. *J. Appl. Physiol.,* 39:457-461, 1975.

26. Huebner, D.E., C.C. Lobeck, and N.R. McSherry. Density and secretory activity of eccrine sweat glands in patients with cystic fibrosis and in healthy controls. *Pediatrics,* 38:613-618, 1966.

27. Inbar, O. *Acclimatization to dry and hot environment in young adults and children 8-10 years old.* Doctoral dissertation, Columbia University, 1978.

28. Inbar, O., O. Bar-Or, R. Dotan, and B. Gutin. Conditioning versus exercise in heat as methods for acclimatizing 8- to 10-year-old boys to dry heat. *J. Appl. Physiol.: Respirat. Environ. Exercise Physiol.,* 50:406-411, 1981.

29. Inbar, O., R. Dotan, O. Bar-Or, and B. Gutin. Heat acclimatization — A comparison between prepubertal boys and young men. *Med. Sci. Sports Exerc.* In press.

30. Inbar, O., R. Dotan, O. Bar-Or, and B. Gutin. *Passive versus active exposures to dry heat as methods for heat acclimatization in prepubertal children.* Submitted for publication.

31. Kessler, W.R., and D.H. Andersen. Heat prostration in fibrocystic disease of the pancreas and other conditions. *Pediatrics,* 8:648-656, 1951.

32. Landing, B.H., T.R. Wells, and M.L. Williamson. "Studies on growth of eccrine sweat glands." In *Human growth, body composition, cell growth, energy, and intelligence,* edited by B.D. Cheek, pp. 382-395, and Appendix 22. Philadelphia: Lea & Febiger, 1968.

33. Leithead, C.S., and A.R. Lind. *Heat stress and heat disorders.* Philadelphia: F.A. Davis, 1964.

34. MacDougall, J.D., P.D. Roche, O. Bar-Or, and J.R. Moroz.

Maximal aerobic capacity of Canadian school children: Prediction based on age-related oxygen cost of running. *Int. J. Sports Med.,* 4:194-198, 1983.

35. Máček, U., J. Vávra, and J. Novosadová. Prolonged exercise in prepubertal boys, I. Cardiovascular & metabolic adjustment. *Europ. J. Appl. Physiol.,* 35:291-298, 1976.

36. Máček, M., J. Vávra, and J. Novosadová. Prolonged exercise in prepubertal boys, II. Changes in plasma volume and in some blood constituents. *Europ. J. Appl. Physiol.,* 35:299-303, 1976.

37. Máčková, J., M. Šturmová, and M. Máček. "Prolonged exercise in prepubertal boys in warm and cold environments." In *Children and Sport,* edited by Y. Ilmarinen and I. Välimäki. Berlin: Springer Verlag, 1984.

38. McConnell, C.M., S. Rostan, and F.A. Puyau. Heat dissipation in children with congenital heart disease. *South Med. J.,* 63:837-841, 1970.

39. McCormick, R.J., and E.R. Buskirk. Heat tolerance of exercising lean and obese middle-aged men. *Fed. Proc.,* 33:441, 1974.

40. Rotstein, A., O. Bar-Or, and R. Dlin. Hemoglobin, hematocrit, and calculated plasma volume changes induced by a short, supramaximal task. *Int. J. Sports Med.,* 3:230-233, 1982.

41. Rowell, L.B. "Cardiovascular adjustments to thermal stress." In *Handbook of physiology. Peripheral circulation and organ blood flow,* edited by J.T. Shephard and F.M. Abboud. Bethesda: Amer. Physiol. Soc. (In print).

42. Shapiro, Y., A. Magazanik, R. Udassin, G. Ben-Baruch, E. Shvartz, and Y. Shoenfeld. Heat intolerance in former heatstroke patients. *Ann Int. Med.,* 90:913-916, 1979.

43. Shattuck, G.C., and M.M. Hilferty. Sunstroke and allied conditions in the United States. *Amer. J. Trop. Med.,* 12:223-245, 1932.

44. Skinner, J.S., O. Bar-Or, V. Bergsteinová, C.W. Bell, D. Royer, and E.R. Buskirk. Comparison of continuous and intermittent tests for determining maximal oxygen intake in children. *Acta Paediatr. Scand. Suppl.* 217:24-28, 1971.

45. Sloan, R.E.G., and W.R. Keatinge. Cooling rates of young people swimming in cold water. *J. Appl. Physiol.,* 35:371-375, 1973.

46. Tanaka, M. Studies on important biological factors influencing the ability to perspire. Part 1. Effect of age on ability to perspire (In Japanese). *J. Physiol. Soc. Japan,* 18:390-394, 1956.

47. Tipton, C.M., and T.K. Tcheng. Iowa wrestling study. Weight loss in high school students. *J. Amer. Med. Assoc.,* 214:1269-1274, 1970.

48. Wagner, J.A., S. Robinson, S.P. Tzankoff, and R.P. Marino. Heat tolerance and acclimatization to work in the heat in relation to age. *J. Appl. Physiol.,* 33:616-622, 1972.

6

Physical Performance
and the Young Diabetic

Yngve Larsson
University Hospital, Linköping, Sweden

Diabetes in children and adolescents is an important pediatric disorder, one in which physical activity can play a crucial role as a therapeutic tool. It can influence the course and prognosis of the disease either positively or negatively, depending on how it is applied. The relationship between diabetes and exercise is of interest not only from the practical, clinical point of view, but also because it illustrates a number of basic physiologic, metabolic, and hemodynamic control systems, many of which have not yet been sufficiently clarified.

Insulin-dependent diabetes mellitus (IDDM), also called type I diabetes, juvenile diabetes, or growth-onset diabetes, is one of the most common chronic disorders among children. Its annual incidence in Northern Europe and North America is about 20 per 100,000 in children from birth to 15 years of age, which corresponds to a prevalence of about 1.5 per 1,000 in children 0-15 years old (11). The question of physical activity among young diabetics is therefore not an isolated clinical issue but a problem that may appear anywhere in society, including families, schools, sports clubs, and working places.

This chapter will review the relations between physical activity and diabetes, with particular reference to diabetes in young people. Although there are rare cases in children of noninsulin dependent diabetes (NIDDM), also called type II diabetes, or maturity onset diabetes in the young (MODY), only the problems occurring in IDDM will be dealt with here. Most of our knowledge in this field is derived either from animal experiments or from studies of IDDM in young adults. For psychological, ethical, and technical reasons there are few studies in children, but in most cases results obtained in studies on young adults in principle are applicable also to children.

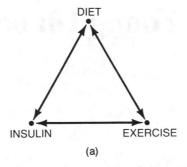

(a)

The Heptagon of Diabetic Control

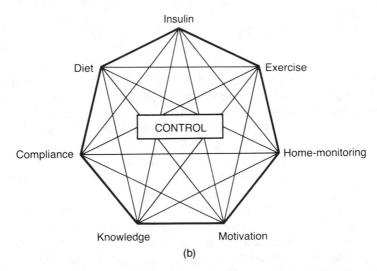

(b)

Figure 6-1. The therapeutic "triad" (Figure 6-1a) in insulin-dependent diabetes mellitus. Therapeutic success, i.e., metabolic control, can be expected only when the triad is supplemented with education, self-care (home-monitoring of blood and urine), motivation, and compliance—The "triad" becomes a "heptagon" (Figure 6-1b).

Physical activity has been recommended in the treatment of diabetes for many years. Even before the discovery of insulin, exercise was said to be beneficial for diabetic patients in promoting their well-being (15). The blood-sugar lowering effect of exercise in insulin-treated patients was first described by Lawrence (35), and since then, particularly through the work of Joslin (39), exercise has been one of the three cornerstones in the treatment of IDDM (Figure 6-1). However, this recommendation was based mostly on general clinical experience with little theoretical justification. Only during the last decade has it become possible to study the problem more systematically, which has led to a greatly increased understanding of the complex mechanisms involved. Exercise should be regarded as a double-edged sword for the IDDM patient, being generally beneficial but having deleterious effects under certain conditions. The benefits must always be weighed against the potential hazards.

Physical activity involves many physiological systems in both diabetics and nondiabetics, the most important of which have been schematically summarized in Figure 6-2. Exercise requires normally functioning cardiovascular, respiratory, gastrointestinal, hepatic, metabolic, hormonal,

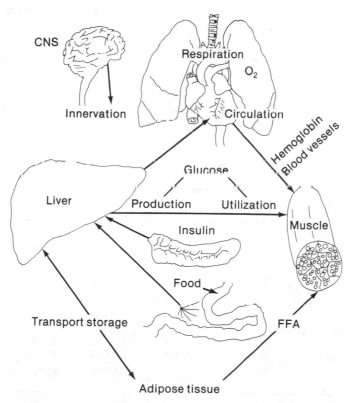

Figure 6-2. A scheme of physiological background factors to exercise in diabetes.

and nervous systems. In IDDM, particular attention must be directed toward metabolism, hormones, and the cardiovascular system.

METABOLIC AND HORMONAL EFFECTS OF EXERCISE

The Nondiabetic Organism

Muscles need oxygen and energy-rich fuel in order to perform mechanical work. Energy is provided through food intake, whereby substrates when not immediately utilized are transferred to the body's different tissue stores. The magnitude of these stores varies with body size, age, and sex. Their approximate dimensions in an adult nonobese male are shown in Table 6-1. The energy contained in circulating substrates, glucose, and free fatty acids (FFA), is a small fraction of the total, and almost all energy is found in tissue depots in the liver, the muscles, and particularly the adipose tissue. Under normal conditions only stores of carbohydrates and lipids are utilized. Combustion of protein would indicate a nonphysiological tissue breakdown.

About 5 kJ/min are utilized in the resting state, but that figure may rise 10- to 20-fold during exercise. At rest, muscle metabolism is almost totally dependent on the oxidation of fatty acids, in contrast to the brain for which glucose is the major fuel both in the resting state and during physical activity.

During exercise, fuel utilization changes significantly depending on the duration and the intensity of the work. For the first few minutes of

Table 6-1

Body Fuel Stores

Substrates	g	kJ	kcal	%
Circulating				
Glucose	20	340	80	
Free fatty acids (FFA)	0.4	16	4	
		356	84	0.05
Tissue depots				
Liver glycogen	85	1500	350	0.2
Muscle glycogen	350	6000	1400	0.8
Muscle protein	6000	105000	25000	15.0
Adipose tissue triglycerides	15000	585000	140000	84.0
		697500	166750	100.0

Modified after Wahren et al. (1978).

muscular activity, energy is derived from the muscles' own glycogen stores through glycogenolysis. As work continues, however, there is an increasing uptake of circulating glucose and FFA, which after about 1 hour's work may be 10 to 30 times above the basal level. Glucose uptake seems to reach a peak after about 2 hours of exercise but FFA utilization continues to increase, which means that in prolonged work lasting 3 or 4 hours or more the relative contribution of fatty acids to muscle energy is about twice that of glucose (Table 6-2).

Fuel utilization during prolonged exercise may consequently be characterized (16) as a triphasic sequence in which glycogen, blood glucose, and FFA successively predominate as the major energy-yielding substrates. The metabolic basis for exhaustion or fatigue is not altogether understood, but it seems to be related to depletion of muscle glycogen, among other factors.

In spite of the large uptake of glucose by the working muscle, the blood glucose level remains normal or decreases only very slightly in moderate or prolonged exercise in nondiabetic subjects. This is explained by hepatic glucose production, which increases almost exactly at the same rate as glucose disappears from the circulation, due to uptake by the working muscles. Hepatic glycogen is the main source of hepatic glucose production, although gluconeogenesis from alanine and other glucose precursors also occurs at an increasing rate with prolonged exer-

Table 6-2

Relative Contributions of Glucose Uptake and Muscle Tissue Fuels to Total Oxygen Uptake in Leg During Prolonged (4 hr.) Mild Exercise

Time (min)		Muscle Tissue Fuels	Glucose Uptake	FFA Uptake	Total Oxygen Uptake
Rest	mmol/min	1.2	0	0	1.2
	%	100	0	0	100
40	mmol/min	5.5	4.1	5.7	15.3
	%	36	27	37	100
90	mmol/min	3.9	7.3	6.5	17.7
	%	22	41	37	100
180	mmol/min	2.5	6.4	8.9	17.7
	%	14	36	50	100
240	mmol/min	1.4	5.4	11.1	17.9
	%	8	30	62	100

Modified from Ahlborg et al. (1974).

cise. Maintaining normoglycemia during exercise is essential for the function of the central nervous system because glucose is the predominant fuel for normal brain function.

Significant hormonal responses also occur during exercise. Plasma insulin drops sharply, while plasma levels of glucagon, the catecholamines, growth hormone, and cortisol all rise. The decrease of insulin is of particular interest. It implies a diminishing of the inhibitory action of insulin on hepatic glycogenolysis, thereby sensitizing the liver to the glycogenolytic action of glucagon and the catecholamines. This facilitates glucose production and the maintenance of a normal blood glucose level. The drop in insulin, which has been demonstrated in children as well as in adults, is accompanied by a simultaneous decrease in the other secretory products of the beta-cell, C-peptide and proinsulin (22).

The fact that there is a high exercise-induced glucose uptake by muscles in spite of insulinopenia suggests that this uptake is perhaps not insulin dependent. However, this hypothesis is contradicted by experiments demonstrating that in the total absence of insulin there is no glucose uptake at all by the working muscle. It has been implied, therefore, that insulin may have a permissive effect in promoting exercise-induced glucose uptake, an effect present even at the low insulin concentrations that are prevalent during exercise. Another explanation could be that although circulating levels of insulin are low, the actual exposure of muscle cells to insulin may be unchanged or even increased because of the greatly augmented blood flow and capillary surface area in the muscle during exercise (55).

The question of possible changes in the concentration and/or affinity of insulin receptors on the target cells is of interest here. It has been shown that exercise in normal young adults induces a significant rise in insulin binding to monocytes, which seems to be associated with an increased insulin sensitivity (30). For technical reasons receptor studies can most easily be done on blood cells, but some studies suggest that the monocyte mirrors quite well the receptor situation of more typical target cells for insulin action, such as the muscle cell (5,19).

Hypoinsulinemia also means a decrease in the antilipolytic effect of insulin, facilitating the release of FFA from adipose tissue and the subsequently increased turnover and oxidation of this important substrate for muscle work, particularly during prolonged exercise. Other factors are also involved in exercise-induced lipolysis, such as an increased beta-adrenergic stimulation.

Immediately after exercise there is a rapid increase in insulin levels, which results in a decrease in hepatic glucose production and a resynthesis of glycogen stores in both liver and muscle. During the immediate postexercise recovery period, plasma FFA levels first remain high or continue to rise and then gradually return to resting levels.

Insulin-Dependent Diabetes Mellitus (IDDM)

In the IDDM patient the effects of exercise are more complex than in the nondiabetic. Deviations from the normal physiological responses described above parallel the prevailing insulin-deficiency and the degree of metabolic control. The effects of exercise in the diabetic must therefore be considered against a background knowledge of the metabolic effects of insulin deprivation, some of which are shown in Figure 6-3. Remember that these effects occur to their full extent only in the totally insulin-deficient organism, such as seen in an experimental animal after surgical or chemical pancreatectomy. In clinical practice it is more common to see less severe degrees of insulin deprivation, but probably every diabetic experiences periods of insufficient metabolic control and varying degrees of insulin deficiency even with vigorous therapeutic efforts.

With regard to muscle glucose uptake, the necessary, minimal, and permissive insulin concentration is practically always present in IDDM patients, either because of some remaining endogenous beta cell secretion or through exogenous insulin treatment. Hence, glucose uptake during exercise is similar to that observed in nondiabetic subjects, and there do not seem to be any significant differences in this regard among patients with good, fair, or poor metabolic control.

However, in most other respects there are important differences between IDDM-patients with and those without adequate metabolic control in regard to the effects of exercise. In patients with poor metabolic control, those who are *ketotic* and hyperglycemic which corresponds in experimental conditions to patients who have been without insulin for at least 24 hours, exercise seems to aggravate the metabolic situation. Glucose production proceeds continuously, unmatched by peripheral glucose uptake, with a consequent further rise in blood glucose, 4-8

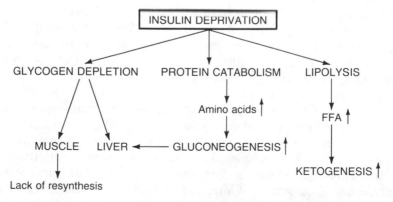

Figure 6-3. Metabolic results of insulin deprivation, of importance in the evaluation of the effects of physical activity in insulin-dependent diabetes.

mmol/l or more above the pre-exercise level. Less glycogen is available in the liver, which increases considerably the gluconeogenesis and amino acid metabolism. Glycogen stores in the liver and muscles are more rapidly utilized and become depleted much sooner than in the normal nondiabetic subjects.

The FFA level in plasma, which is already elevated at rest in such patients, continues to rise during exercise. The concomitant high muscle uptake of FFA may be more than twice a large as the FFA uptake seen in nondiabetic patients. Ketone bodies, which in the nondiabetic are present in plasma in very low concentrations and not utilized as fuel by the muscles, are moderately elevated at rest in the insulin-deficient ketotic diabetic. During exercise the production of ketone bodies is markedly accelerated, leading to a pronounced ketonemia. Although a certain percentage of the ketone bodies are utilized by the muscles, this does not prevent an aggravation of the diabetic condition, a sustained postexercise ketonemia, and possibly even ketoacidosis. In such patients exercise may therefore provoke a severe catabolic situation even after a relatively short time, a condition seen in the normal nondiabetic subject only after several hours of prolonged heavy work.

In *nonketotic*, normoglycemic, or mildly hyperglycemic, insulin-treated IDDM patients the effects of exercise are completely different. In such patients exercise does not aggravate the metabolic state but, on the contrary, has a beneficial effect. It decreases blood glucose levels which may become completely normal. Liver and muscle glycogen stores are not depleted, and postexercise glycogen synthesis may even take place at a higher rate than normal. FFA and ketone body production are equal to or only slightly above normal levels. In diabetic patients, maintained normoglycemic through continuous insulin infusion, exercise does not seem to cause any metabolic alterations other than those seen in non-diabetic subjects.

In the well controlled, nonketotic diabetic patient, however, there is a certain risk of exercise-induced *hypoglycemia*. The drop in insulin levels that normally occurs during exercise (see above) is not present, and hepatic glucose output may therefore be suppressed by insulin below the level necessary to match peripheral glucose uptake.

The degree of insulinemia in the IDDM patient is determined by the gradual absorption of the injected insulin from the subcutaneous depot. The absorption profile is related to the type of insulin preparation used, whether short-acting or long-acting. The risk of hypoglycemia is particularly noticeable if exercise takes place simultaneously with the peak action of the injected insulin. Furthermore, several studies have shown that the rate of absorption of injected insulin may be accelerated by exercise, particularly if insulin has been injected in a limb, such as the leg, which is involved in the physical activity (7,30). Increased blood flow is the most likely explanation for this change in absorption, which may often unexpectedly contribute to a hypoglycemic reaction.

However, exercise-induced hypoglycemia can in most cases be prevented by glucose or carbohydrate ingestion immediately before exercise. The effect of such intake is particularly beneficial because carbohydrates ingested in connection with physical activity often escape hepatic retention and are therefore immediately available for raising blood glucose and for utilization by the working muscles (53).

Some of the most important metabolic effects of exercise have been summarized in Tables 6-3 and 6-4, as they occur in nondiabetics (ND), nonketotic, fairly well controlled IDDM patients (NKD) and in ketotic, insulin-deficient IDDM patients (KD). In conclusion, it is obvious that exercise has a beneficial normalizing effect in young IDDM patients when their diabetes is in good metabolic control and their insulin administration is optimal. By contrast, insulin-deficient patients in poor metabolic control run the risk that exercise may seriously aggravate their diabetic state.

CIRCULATORY EFFECTS
OF EXERCISE AND PHYSICAL FITNESS

Healthy Children

The physiological adaptations taking place during acute physical activity are well known and have been extensively described in the relevant literature (4). In brief, exercise is accompanied by increased sympathetic

Table 6-3

Relative Contributions of Substrates
to Total Oxygen Uptake in Leg After 40 min
of Moderately Heavy Exercise in Nondiabetics (ND),
Nonketotic Diabetics (NKD), and Ketotic Diabetics (KD)

		Muscle Tissue Fuels	Glucose Uptake	FFA Uptake	Ketone Body Uptake	Total Oxygen Uptake
ND	mmol/min	25.7	13.4	14.4	0	53.5
	%	48	25	27	0	100
NKD	mmol/min	18.8	13.4	16.3	1.0	49.5
	%	38	27	33	2	100
KD	mmol/min	4.2	15.6	29.0	3.1	51.9
	%	8	30	56	6	100

Modified from Wahren et al. (1978).

Table 6-4

**A Simplified Summary of the Effects of Exercise
in Nondiabetics (ND), Nonketotic Diabetics (NKD),
and Ketotic Diabetics (KD)**

		ND	NKD	KD
Blood	Glucose	(−)	−	+ +
	FFA	+	+ +	+ + +
	Ketones	+	+ +	+ + +
Muscle	Glucose uptake	+	+	+
	FFA uptake	+	+	+ + +
	Ketones uptake	0	+	+ + +
	Postexercise glycogen synthesis	+ + +	+ + +	+
Liver	Glucose output	+	+	+
	Glycogenolysis	+	+ +	+ +
	Gluconeogenesis	(+)	+ +	+ + +
	Ketones production	0	+	+ + +

− = decrease
+, + +, + + + = varying degrees of increment
0 = nonexistent

tone, heart rate (2-4 times), cardiac output, and blood pressure, with a decreased plasma volume. Dilatation of muscle vessles and vasoconstriction of vessels in the kidney and splanchnic area leads to a complete change in blood distribution, with an increase of muscle flow from about 20% to about 75% of the cardiac output, at the expense of almost all other tissues except the brain and heart (Table 6-5). There is a marked increase in oxygen uptake and pulmonary ventilation.

All these changes occur with a great degree of individual variation, depending on sex, age, body dimensions, body composition (particularly the relationship between body fat and lean body mass), and the nature of the work including its intensity and duration. Furthermore, training and psychological factors (e.g., attitudes and motivation) influence the physiological responses to exercise. Taken together these factors determine the physical fitness of each individual. In practical and clinical work when an objective measure of such fitness is needed standardized exercise tests are helpful. A multistage bicycle ergometry test (17,52) is often used for children, in which the child is exposed to stepwise increasing work loads while heart rate, respiration, blood pressure, oxygen consumption, or other variables are simultaneously being measured and recorded. The work load increment may be 0.2 to 0.5 Watt per kg body weight and the duration of each work period may be 3 to 6 minutes. For healthy children a work load of 1.0, 1.5, and 2.0 W/kg corresponds to

Table 6-5

Relative Distribution of Cardiac Output to Organ Systems at Rest and at Three Levels of Physical Exercise (After Horvath)

	At Rest	Light	During Exercise Moderate	Heavy
Cardiac output l/min	5.8	9.5	17.5	25.0
Distribution to organs (%)				
Heart	4.3	3.7	4.3	4.0
Brain	12.9	7.9	4.3	3.0
Muscle	20.7	47.4	71.4	88.0
Skin	8.6	15.8	10.9	2.4
Kidney	19.0	9.5	3.4	1.0
Splanchnic	25.9	11.6	3.4	1.2
Other	8.6	4.2	2.3	0.4

light, moderate, and heavy exercise, respectively, or approximately 25-35%, 50-60%, and 70-80% of the maximal working capacity; that is the maximal quantity of oxygen (max $\dot{V}O_2$) that can be taken up in the lungs during exercise close to the point of exhaustion.

Max $\dot{V}O_2$ may be used as a measure of fitness. In healthy children it varies between 40-60 ml/kg/min in boys and 35-50 ml/kg/min in girls. Expressed in l/min it amounts to 1-2 l/min for children 5-10 years old and 2-3 l/min for youths 10-20 years old. Peak values of 3.5 l/min for boys and 2.5 l/min for girls occur at 18-20 years of age. After 20 years of age there is no further rise in max $\dot{V}O_2$ and a gradual decline begins at about age 30. Before puberty there is no significant difference between boys and girls, but during puberty max $\dot{V}O_2$ is higher in males than in females, a difference seen throughout life.

For routine clinical purposes the determination of max $\dot{V}O_2$ is cumbersome and inconvenient and fitness may instead be estimated by determining heart rates (in steady state) at different submaximal workloads. The workload corresponding to a heart rate of 170 beats/min (W_{170}) can be calculated and used for intra-individual comparisons and also, although with less accuracy, for comparisons between children of the same age. A useful nomogram has been constructed (3) for estimating max $\dot{V}O_2$ from the pulse rate at a certain submaximal workload. The maximal heart rate attainable during exercise decreases with age. At about 10 years of age it is about 210 beats/min and decreases thereafter about 10 beats per decade (rule of thumb: $HR_{max} = 220 - age$). A complementary method by which an individual's subjective perception of exertion in an exercise test can be rated (RPE) has been introduced by Borg (9). Changes in RPE correlate well with changes in heart rate.

Young Diabetics

The considerably increased demands on the cardiovascular system during physical exercise raise the question of whether the young insulin-treated IDDM-patient should exercise in the same way as healthy children, considering the higher potential long-term vulnerability of the diabetic's cardiovascular system. There are relatively few studies of the physical fitness of young IDDM patients. In Sweden, interest in this subject began in the 1960s with a study by Larsson et al. (34), in which the physical working capacity (PWC) was studied in a group of 22 diabetic girls, ages 10-18, who had been diabetic for 1 to 4 years. For comparison 27 nondiabetic control girls of similar age were also studied. While there was no difference in PWC between the 10- to 12-year-old diabetic and nondiabetic girls, a difference was found in the 13- to 14-year-olds and an even greater one in the 15- to 18-year-old girls. The diabetic patients in the adolescent group had a significantly higher pulse rate than the controls at the same work load.

A similar study was later conducted by Sterky (48) in diabetic children, both boys and girls. He confirmed that the heart rate at fixed work loads tended to be higher in diabetic than in nondiabetic children. The difference became more evident when physical fitness was expressed as heart rate at a work load of 10 kpm/kg/min (1.6 W/kg/min). When max $\dot{V}O_2$ was calculated with the help of the nomogram mentioned above, it was also found that the diabetics had a lower max $\dot{V}O_2$ expressed as ml/kg than the nondiabetics. The differences were more pronounced among boys than girls and also more obvious in diabetics who had had the condition since early childhood. After puberty and with increasing age, diabetic children of both sexes showed a tendency to deviate more and more from the corresponding nondiabetics.

In both these studies (34,48) the lower physical fitness of the diabetics was explained as the result of inadequate training and low degree of participation in physical education at school. Rutenfranz et al. (45) similarly found a lower PWC in German adolescent diabetics but not in younger diabetic children. Furthermore, in a more recent study Baran and Dorchy (6) found that 33 diabetic boys, age 11-17 years, had a significantly lower PWC than nondiabetic Belgian boys of similar age, both when expressed as W/kg or as max $\dot{V}O_2$ (ml/kg/min).

On the other hand, Elö et al. (12) and Hagan et al. (21) did not find any differences between diabetic and nondiabetic children with regard to cardiorespiratory responses to maximal and submaximal work. However, in their studies the children were younger and had had diabetes for a shorter period of time than in the previous studies mentioned above.

TRAINING OF YOUNG DIABETICS

Effects on Work Capacity

The suggestion (34,48) that the observed lower PWC of diabetic children and adolescents is due to lack of training led to studies of the effects of physical training programs for such patients. Larsson et al. (34) showed that the working capacity of diabetic girls increased after both a 2-month moderate training program and a shorter, more strenuous 1-week training at a winter camp. The increase was most evident in the 13- to 14-year-old girls but less marked both in the 10- to 12-year-olds and in the 15- to 18-year-olds. As the intensity of training in this study was relatively moderate, another study was made by the same group (32) in which the effects of a much more intense physical training program were studied in 6 diabetic boys, ages 15 to 19, and 6 matched nondiabetic boys of the same age. The mean duration of diabetes was 7.3 years (range 4-12 years) and the mean insulin dose was 71 units per 24 hours, given in split doses twice a day to all patients. There were no symptoms or signs of diabetic angiopathy in any of the patients. These 12 boys, who all had been selected because of a previously expressed interest in sports, submitted to a rigorous 5-month training program conducted by a teacher in physical education. At the same time they were under continuous medical supervision and repeated tests were made of their PWC at submaximal work loads. The program concluded with a national cross-country ski race ("Vasaloppet"), covering a distance of about 25 to 30 km per day for three consecutive days (total distance = 85 km).

At the beginning of the study, the physical fitness of the diabetic boys was slightly below that of the nondiabetic boys, confirming the results of the previous studies mentioned above. At the end of the training, a highly significant improvement of about 30-35% had taken place in both groups of boys. Their PWC was then comparable to that of well trained athletes (Table 6-6), the mean $\dot{V}O_2$ being 42 ml/kg/min for the diabetics (range 31-51) and 47 ml/kg/min for the nondiabetics (range 37-51). However, although the performance values in individual, exceptional diabetic boys were above those of some of the nondiabetic boys, the diabetics as a group had values slightly below the nondiabetics. Thus, even a very rigorous training program did not completely equalize the two groups.

In a later study (42) a comparison was made between 7 physically very active and well trained diabetic boys, mean age 17.3 years (range 16-19) and 5 nondiabetic boys, mean age 16.3 years (range 13-18), who participated in regular endurance training as members of a bicycle club. These 12 subjects were studied during a 60-min. exercise period on a

Table 6-6

Effects on Physical Performance of a 5-Month Rigorous Training Program in 6 Diabetic and 6 Nondiabetic Boys

| | Diabetics | | | Nondiabetics | | |
	b.	a.	Change %	b.	a.	Change %
Heart rate (beats/min) at 900 kpm/min (147 W)	178	157	− 11.8	171	148	− 13.5
Heart rate (beats/min) at maximal workload	199	191	− 4.0	201	189	− 6.0
Maximal oxygen uptake (liters)	2.33	3.08	+ 32.2	2.55	3.33	+ 30.6
PWC$_{170}$ (Watt/min)	139	183	+ 31.7	148	198	+ 33.8

b. = before training
a. = after training
PWC$_{170}$ = calculated workload at a heart rate of 170/min
After Larsson et al., 1964a (32).

bicycle ergometer at an average intensity of 63.3% (diabetics) and 57.8% (nondiabetics) of their maximal working capacity. Again it was found that the mean max $\dot{V}O_2$ was significantly higher in the nondiabetics than in the diabetics, being 61 ml/kg/min (range 55-70) and 54 ml/kg/min (range 48-66), respectively. Heart rate and the systolic blood pressure during the test increased significantly more in the diabetic than in the nondiabetic boys. The RPE according to the Borg scale (see above) was also determined. It was highly correlated with heart rate and relative work load, and in this regard no differences between diabetics and nondiabetics were seen.

In summary, these studies have shown that diabetic children and adolescents often have a lower PWC than healthy children, that they can improve their fitness by regular training programs, but that they do not seem able as a group to reach the same average level of physical performance capacity as nondiabetic subjects. This does not exclude exceptional young diabetics from becoming top athletes and even reaching the championship level in sports competition. There are several well known examples of such diabetics.

Specific factors may prevent the average diabetic from getting the same full advantage of training programs as the nondiabetic. Some muscle enzyme activities are age-dependent and may also be influenced by training (14). The glycolytic enzyme phosphofructokinase, and the oxidative enzyme succinate-dehydrogenase, for example, have not yet been studied in diabetic children. Nor is it known whether work-induced muscle hypertrophy may in some way be impeded in the physically active IDDM patient. Considering the breakdown of proteins and general wasting that is characteristic of the diabetic organism (18), and the well known effect of insulin on growth, one cannot rule out that the relative insulin deficiency that exists even in well controlled cases may prevent the diabetics from getting the same muscle hypertrophy during physical training as the nondiabetic.

Likewise, little is known about muscle fiber composition in IDDM. Saltin et al. (46) did not find any differences in the relative distribution of slow and fast fiber types in a group of 8 adult IDDM patients, ages 23-45, in comparison to age-matched healthy subjects. It is not known, however, whether the changes that normally occur in the fiber population during and after physical exercise are different in IDDM patients than in nondiabetic subjects (23,44). Saltin et al. (46) showed that the increased capillarization that is a normal response to exercise (2) did not occur to the same extent in 8 IDDM patients. Wallberg-Henriksson et al. (55) have also found evidence that muscle capillary density fails to increase in type I diabetes during training. This may be a sign of early diabetic angiopathy, related to diabetic membrane thickening. Peterson et al. (43), however, have shown a decreased muscle capillary basement membrane thickening in 7 IDDM patients after an 8- to 10-month exercise program, although this also included systematic attempts to normalize blood glucose.

Effects on Diabetic Control

In contrast to the obvious metabolic effects of *acute* exercise described above the metabolic effects of *long-term* physical training in IDDM are less distinct. There have also been relatively few systematic studies of this matter. One difficulty is the problem of agreeing on the definition of good or adequate metabolic control and on the criteria to use in assessing diabetic control. Another problem in long-term studies of diabetics is the difficulty of isolating the effect of one factor, such as physical training, from all other variables that may influence diabetic control during a prolonged period of time.

However, some studies support the general clinical experience that diabetic children who are physically active have lower blood glucose levels, lower glycosylated hemoglobin values, less glucosuria, and a more stable metabolism than diabetic children who are more sedentary. At camps for diabetic children these observations have been repeatedly confirmed. Thus, Larsson et al. (33,34) in the studies mentioned above showed that the glucosuria index (the frequency of aglucosuric urine tests) more than doubled during the period of high physical activity—in spite of a markedly increased caloric intake. This increase was about 45% for girls and 70% for boys. Similarly, Dahl-Jørgensen et al. (10) demonstrated a significant decrease of glycosylated hemoglobin (HbA$_1$) in 14 diabetic children, ages 9 to 15, who participated in a supervised exercise program for 5 months. Ludvigsson (36) calculated an activity index based on the patients' own recording of their physical activities during one ordinary week and found a significant correlation between this index and the glucosuria index, such as used by Larsson et al. (33,34).

An improvement in glucose tolerance has been demonstrated in adult IDDM patients by Maehlum & Pruett (38), while Wallberg-Henriksson et al. (55) have more recently shown a significant increase in insulin-stimulated glucose uptake in IDDM patients after a 16-week training period. This would indicate that training has an effect, possibly receptor mediated (41), on insulin sensitivity and glucose tolerance in IDDM patients similar to that seen in obesity (8) and chemical diabetes (NIDDM) in middle-age subjects (47). Nondiabetic athletes have 69% higher insulin binding to monocytes than sedentary control subjects, and physical training of the latter resulted in a 35% rise in insulin binding to monocytes (31).

Effects on Blood Lipids

In contrast to the consistent changes of plasma FFA during acute exercise (described above), long-term effects of physical training on blood lipids and lipid metabolism in IDDM are much less evident. Considering the accepted relationships between a sedentary life and hyperlipemia, obesity, cardiovascular diseases, and glucose tolerance in the adult nondiabetic population, it may seem surprising that there are relatively few systematic studies in young IDDM patients of the effects of training on lipid metabolism.

Hyperlipemia is common in insulin-deficient, ketotic IDDM patients but rare in insulin-treated diabetic children, whose average blood lipid levels may be slightly above those of nondiabetic children but still within normal limits (49). During periods of increased physical activity, serumlipids tend to fall in both diabetic and nondiabetic children (33). This is true for serum cholesterol, phospholipids, and triglycerides. In adult IDDM patients a decrease of cholesterol with a simultaneous increase of HDL-cholesterol has been described (20). This is of particular interest because of the negative correlation between HDL cholesterol and cardiovascular disease. Studies of the HDL cholesterol levels in physically active versus sedentary diabetic children have not yet been done, but they are obviously needed.

In spite of the inadequacy of present knowledge in this field it seems reasonable to conclude that, by and large, regular physical activity should have the same beneficial effects on lipid metabolism in diabetic as in nondiabetic children and adolescents, that is, helping to prevent hyperlipemia and obesity and possibly helping to prevent cardiovascular disease.

EXERCISE AND DIABETIC MICROANGIOPATHY

Microangiopathy is the most serious complication of childhood diabetes. Its main manifestations are diabetic retinopathy which in the advanced stage may cause poor vision, nephropathy with gradual loss of renal function leading to hypertension and uremia, generalized atherosclerosis which may cause premature coronary heart disease, cerebrovascular disease, and/or gangrene. Another common complication is neuropathy with a mixed vascular and metabolic etiology, which affects the peripheral motor and sensory nerves as well as the autonomic nervous system.

Clinical symptoms and signs of microangiopathy do not usually appear until the patients have had diabetes for more than 15 or 20 years and are no longer pediatric patients. However, recent studies indicate that subclinical, asymptomatic, functional, vascular, and neurological abnormalities may be present much earlier (29). Of great importance is the clinical and experimental evidence of a close association between these early lesions and hyperglycemia. Strict control of the blood glucose level may therefore prevent or postpone the later appearance of permanent, irreversible vascular disease.

A logical question is whether physical activity, training, and sports have a positive or negative influence on the development of microangiopathy. If normoglycemia protects against diabetic vascular disease then the blood glucose-lowering effect of exercise in the adequately insulin-treated young diabetic must be regarded as a potentially important factor in the prevention of microangiopathy. It is also probable that the hemodynamic effects of regular exercise benefit the cardiovascular system by increasing cardiac output, improving blood flow, and facilitating oxygen transport. The blood lipid-lowering effect of exercise should also help preserve the integrity of the vascular system and protect the arteries of the young diabetic against premature atherosclerosis. If regular exercise helps prevent obesity in IDDM patients, this too might decrease the risk of vascular disease.

However, possible negative factors must be considered. When vascular lesions are present, even if not yet clinically manifest, the value of exercise may be questioned. The increase in blood pressure which accompanies short periods of exercise, and which may be more exaggerated in diabetics than in nondiabetics (28,42), may have a harmful influence on vessels already damaged by early angiopathy, especially in the eye, kidney, or heart. Of particular interest is asymptomatic autonomic neuropathy, a condition characterized by decreased cardiac beat-to-beat variation during forced respiration, orthostatic hypotension, and decreased spontaneous variation of blood flow in the feet (24,51). Such patients have abnormal hemodynamic responses during exercise and do not tolerate work load as well as diabetics without neuropathy (25).

Another early abnormality in some diabetics is increased glomerular albumin leakage into the urine. Exercise seems to provoke an increase of such leakage in some patients (27,40), particularly in those with poor metabolic control. Whether this sign of early renal dysfunction is related to long-term diabetic nephropathy is not clear, but it represents a vascular abnormality that is aggravated by exercise.

In conclusion, it is probably true with regard to microangiopathy that in the great majority of diabetic children and adolescents the advantages of physical exercise outweigh the possible negative effects. If there is any doubt, particularly for adolescents who have had diabetes for more than 10 years, it is prudent to have a careful medical evaluation of the cardiovascular system before recommending a heavy training program. Once microangiopathy has become symptomatic and clinically manifest, exercise may be harmful and should then be undertaken with great caution. This is rarely a pediatric problem; most IDDM patients in this situation have reached maturity.

CLINICAL IMPLICATIONS
AND PSYCHOSOCIAL ASPECTS

It is clear from the foregoing discussion that muscular work, that is, physical activity and exercise, is an important and sometimes very powerful tool in the treatment of young diabetics. However, it should only be used in close combination with the other components of the diabetic therapy: insulin, diet, and education (Figure 6-1). It is important that the patients understand that exercise cannot replace insulin in the treatment of IDDM and that its beneficial effects cannot be fully utilized unless the diabetic stage is adequately controlled with insulin. Young diabetic patients and their families need thorough and often repeated instruction on these relationships.

Ideally, all diabetic children and adolescents should have a daily physical exercise program, regularly scheduled in relation to insulin injections and meals in such a way that the beneficial blood glucose-lowering effect of muscular work is maximally utilized without leading to hypoglycemia. But this ideal situation is not always realized.

In spite of all the evidence of the value of physical exercise for young IDDM patients, it is still a part of the treatment that tends to be neglected in clinical practice. The few pages spent on exercise in most textbooks on diabetes, in comparison with the extensive chapters on insulin and diet, may be taken as evidence of this statement. The fact that the average physical fitness of diabetic teenagers, because of lack of training, is lower than that of nondiabetics of the same age, sex, and size seems to be another confirmation of this therapeutic neglect.

There are several possible explanations for this. In contrast to insulin and diet, exercise cannot easily be measured and prescribed in fixed quantities. Furthermore, diabetic children have been prevented from participating in physical education in school, as was shown by Sterky (48) among diabetic schoolchildren in Stockholm in 1960-1961, probably due to an erroneous belief of parents, teachers, health workers, or the children themselves that they are sick and therefore, like children with some other chronic diseases, should be exempted from physical activities. However, in most countries this misconception probably no longer prevails.

A more common reason for insufficient physical exercise in the daily life of many young IDDM patients is the fear of exercise-induced hypoglycemia, not uncommon among doctors, nurses, and other health workers as well as among the parents and children. This fear is often based on real experience, since exercise-induced hypoglycemia does occur, often unnecessarily, due to an insufficient energy supply in relation to the intensity and duration of the work. Hypoglycemia is the most important limiting factor for adolescent diabetics when performing prolonged heavy work (32), and diabetics are therefore more dependent on a liberal carbohydrate intake before and during exercise than nondiabetics. It is also important to know that exogenous glucose consumed in connection with exercise is preferentially utilized by the working muscles (53). All this is a matter of education; patients and parents must learn that hypoglycemia in connection with exercise can be prevented in almost all situations if the food intake before and during the work period is adequate.

In planning physical activities, due consideration should be paid to the diabetic's meals and insulin treatment. Exercise-induced hypoglycemia seems to be less frequent in metabolically well-controlled diabetic children with a near normal blood glucose level than in cases with so-called brittle diabetics who have large glycemic fluctuations. Preliminary experience also indicates that continuous insulin infusion by pump treatment, which leads to a more or less normoglycemic state, seems to make exercise-induced hypoglycemia disappear in patients who are liable to develop such reactions when on conventional treatment.

During periods of increased physical activity, whether of short or prolonged duration, the basic principle of management should be to increase the energy intake without changing the insulin dose. A moderate reduction of the insulin dose may be acceptable only when the tendency to hypoglycemia persists in spite of increased energy intake and when the activity level is expected to be high for a relatively prolonged period of time, such as may occur during the long holidays, at camps, or during periods of intense physical training. In order to prevent a "rebound" effect and a deterioration of the metabolic control at the end of the active period, patients should reduce their food intake as soon as the additional energy is no longer required, such as when returning home after a camp stay.

In diabetic children and adolescents, spontaneous motivation for exercise is of course crucially important. If they lack this it is extremely difficult to make them physically active. Medical staff, parents, and others should be careful not to remind the young diabetics too often and persistently about the need for exercise, as this may have the adverse effect of making exercise a necessary evil, part of an obnoxious therapeutic program. This has to some extent been supported by the results of a study of the attitudes of juvenile diabetics towards physical exercise (37). Although the majority of the patients in this study knew and understood the importance of physical exercise, many of them found it difficult to convert theory into practical compliant behavior. In this regard patients need support and positive stimulation without nagging.

Diabetic children and adolescents do not differ from other children concerning their basic interest and motivation for physical activity. Some like it but others do not. The diabetic child's interest in exercise reflects that of the whole family. One cannot expect a child to be physically active if the rest of the family leads a sedentary life. In such cases therapeutic efforts should aim at changing the lifestyle of the whole family. Such attempts should of course be flexible, and individual variations with regard to regularity and persistence in exercise must be accepted.

Before puberty, diabetic children rarely have a problem in this regard, as they have a natural inclination to be physically active and as a rule are almost constantly on the move. This probably explains why, as mentioned earlier, there are no great differences in PWC between diabetic and nondiabetic children before puberty. Difficulties may arise thereafter, however, as shown by the gradually increasing average difference in physical fitness between diabetic and nondiabetic adolescents. Although a decline in the average amount of physical activity occurs in most teenagers between 15 to 20 years of age, at least in Sweden according to a study by Engström (13) this decline seems to be more evident in diabetic teenagers. This is probably due to changes in their social situation, new interests in connection with maturity and puberty, and an increasing awareness of their handicap. Television, automobiles, reading, and further education are also strong competitors with physical activities in the lives of adolescents, whether diabetic or nondiabetic. Opportunities for competition in sports also become less frequent. The inclination of many sports programs to give priority to championship athletes may assume certain blame in this regard as it may have a disheartening effect on many physically less talented young people.

The problem of how to create an interest in exercise for less motivated young diabetics remains a challenge for everybody in some way concerned with such patients. It is a question of how to utilize and develop the interest in exercise which by nature exists in every person (50). All means should be tried on an individual basis, with flexibility for age, sex, interests, family habits, and social situation. The ideal of a daily regular exercise program may not always be attained, but even an irregular program may be beneficial. However, occasional short spells of intense activity between long sedentary periods are much less effective with regard to both fitness and metabolic control than is a lighter but more consistent endurance training program. Many diabetics feel it helpful to keep a diary of their daily physical activities and they should be encouraged to do so.

The choice of activities is not as important, as there is no indication that any particular type of exercise may be preferable to another for young diabetics. Walking, running, swimming, cycling, skating, rowing, ball games (e.g., football, tennis, badminton) or dancing — all are acceptable if enjoyable by the diabetic child or adolescent. Participation in sports competition should also be permitted as long as it is preceded by careful and well planned training. The support obtained through different kinds of group activity is a stimulation that may encourage many diabetic adolescents to start an exercise program. Finally, it should be emphasized that one important effect of regular physical activity, an effect that every young diabetic ought to experience, is the sense of well-being that it gives. To be successful in physical performance, to enjoy the pleasant feeling of normal fatigue after an active day, creates self-confidence and replaces the feeling of being handicapped.

Regular exercise with a concomitant high level of physical fitness thus adds quality to the life of young diabetics and helps them remain healthy in adult life. The statement that man was not meant to be a sedentary animal is true for diabetics as well as for nondiabetics.

SUMMARY

1. Exercise has a beneficial normalizing effect in insulin-dependent diabetic children and adolescents only when their diabetes is in good metabolic control and insulin administration is optimal. Insulin-deficient patients in poor metabolic control, on the other hand, run the risk that exercise may seriously aggravate their diabetic state.

2. The physical working capacity of diabetic children and adolescents is often lower than that of healthy children, but the physical fitness of the young diabetics can be improved by regular training programs. But for reasons not yet clear they do not as a group seem able to reach the same average level of physical performance capacity as comparable non-

diabetic subjects, although there are individual exceptions to this general rule.

3. Regular physical activity improves diabetic control in young insulin-treated diabetics and leads to lower blood glucose levels, lower glycosylated hemoglobin values, less glucosuria, and a more stable metabolism in spite of an often markedly increased caloric intake. Simultaneously, a normalization of blood lipids takes place.

4. Exercise-induced hypoglycemia may occur in the well controlled, nonketotic diabetic patient and is due to suppression of hepatic glucose output in response to an abnormal insulinemia. Such hypoglycemia is the most important limiting factor for adolescent diabetics when performing prolonged heavy work. However, it can usually be prevented by a liberal carbohydrate intake before and during the exercise period.

5. To fully utilize the beneficial effects of physical exercise, the young diabetics and their families need thorough and often repeated expert instruction on the interrelationships between insulin, food intake, and muscular work.

6. The psychosocial effects of regular physical activity are of great value for motivated young diabetics, giving them an increased sense of well-being and self-confidence and dispelling feelings of being handicapped. However, many diabetics lack the attitude and the motivation for a physically active life. Health workers therefore should try harder to interest young diabetics in participating in physical activity programs.

7. Although exercise may help prevent the development of long-term diabetic microangiopathy and neuropathy by improving metabolic control, lowering blood lipids, and increasing circulatory dimensions, the value of exercise is less obvious once the signs of such microangiopathy or neuropathy have appeared. In such cases exercise may be harmful for the diabetic and should be undertaken with great caution and only after careful medical evaluation.

8. In conclusion, exercise is a most important part of the treatment of young diabetics, both for short-term metabolic control and for prevention of long-term complications, but it may be harmful if practiced (a) when diabetic control is poor, (b) if the patient does not know how to prevent hypoglycemia, and (c) if there is a manifest major vascular complication or neuropathy.

REFERENCES

1. Ahlborg, G., P. Felig, L. Hagenfeldt, R. Hendler, and J. Wahren. Substrate turnover during prolonged exercise in man. *J. Clin. Invest.*, 53:1080-1090, 1974.

2. Andersen, P., and J. Henriksson. Capillary supply of the quadriceps femoris of man: Adaptive response to exercise. *J. Physiol.*, 270:677-690, 1977.

3. Åstrand, I. Aerobic work capacity in men and women with special reference to age. *Acta Physiol. Scand.,* 49 (suppl.):169, 1960.

4. Åstrand, P.O., and K. Rodahl. *Textbook of work physiology — physiological bases of exercise* (2nd ed.). New York: McGraw-Hill, 1977.

5. Bar, R.S., P. Gorden, J. Roth, C.R. Kahn, and P. De Meyts. Fluctuation in the affinity and concentration of insulin receptors on circulating monocytes of obese patients. *J. Clin. Invest.,* 58:1123-1135, 1976.

6. Baran, D. and H. Dorchy. Aptitude physique de l'adolescent diabétique. *Bull. Europ. Physiopath. Resp.,* 18:51-58, 1982.

7. Berger, M., P.A. Halban, J.P. Assal, R.E. Offord, M. Vranic, and A.E. Renold. Pharmacokinetics of subcutaneously injected tritiated insulin: Effects of exercise. *Diabetes,* 28 (suppl.), 1:53-57, 1979.

8. Björntorp, P., G. Holm, B. Jacobsson, K. Schillder-de-Jounge, P.-A. Lundberg, L. Sjöström, U. Smith, and L. Sullivan. Physical training in human hyperplastic obesity. IV. Effects on the hormonal status. *Metabolism,* 26:319-328, 1977.

9. Borg, G. Perceived exertion as an indicator of somatic stress. *Scand. J. Rehab. Med.,* 2:92-98, 1970.

10. Dahl-Jørgensen, K., H.D. Meen, Kr.F. Hanssen, and Ø. Aagenaes. The effect of exercise on diabetic control and hemoglobin A₁ (HbA₁) in children. *Acta Paediatr. Scand. Suppl.,* 283:53-56, 1980.

11. Dahlquist, G., K.H. Gustavsson, G. Holmgren, B. Hägglöf, Y. Larsson, K.O. Nilsson, G. Samuelson, G. Sterky, B. Thalme, and S. Wall. The incidence of diabetes mellitus in Swedish children 0-14 years of age. A prospective study 1977-1980. *Acta Paediatr. Scand.,* 71:7-14, 1982.

12. Elö, O., L. Hirvonen, T. Peltonen, and I. Valimaki. Physical working capacity of normal and diabetic children. *Ann. Paediat. Fenn.,* 11:25-31, 1965.

13. Engström, L.-M. Physical activity of children and youth. *Acta Paediatr. Scand. Suppl.,* 283:101-105, 1980.

14. Eriksson, B.O. Physical training, oxygen supply and muscle metabolism in 11- to 13-year-old boys. *Acta Physiol. Scand.,* 86 (suppl.):384, 1972.

15. Errebo-Knudsen, E.O. Diabetes mellitus and exercise. A physiopathological study of muscular work in patients with diabetes mellitus. *Reports of the Steno Memorial Hospital,* 3:1-148, 1948.

16. Felig, P., and J. Wahren. Fuel homeostasis in exercise. *N. Engl. J. Med.,* 293:1078-1084, 1975.

17. Godfrey, S. *Exercise testing in children. Applications in health and disease.* London: Saunders, 1974.

18. Goldberg, A. Influence of insulin and contractile activity on muscle size and protein balance. *Diabetes,* 28 (suppl.), 1:18-24, 1979.

19. Gorden, P. Hormone receptor interactions. *Diabetes,* 28 (suppl), 1:8-12, 1979.

20. Gunnarsson, R., H. Wallberg-Henriksson, J. Henriksson, J. Östman, and J. Wahren. "Exercise and physical training in type I diabetes." In *Recent trends in diabetes research*, edited by H. Boström and N. Ljungstedt. Stockholm: Skandia International Symposium, Almqvist & Wiksell International, 1982.

21. Hagan, R.D., J.F. Marks, and P.A. Warren. Physiologic responses of juvenile-onset diabetic boys to muscular work. *Diabetes*, 28:114-119, 1979

22. Heding, L.G., and J. Ludvigsson. B-cell response to exercise in diabetic and non-diabetic children. *Acta Paediatr. Scand. Suppl.*, 283:57-61, 1980.

23. Henriksson, K.G. Muscle histochemistry and muscle function. *Acta Paediatr. Scand. Suppl.*, 283:15-19, 1980.

24. Hilsted, J., H. Galbo, and N.J. Christensen. Cardiovascular, hormonal and metabolic responses to graded exercise in juvenile diabetics with and without autonomic neuropathy. *Acta Paediatr. Scand. Suppl.*, 283:95-100, 1980.

25. Hilsted, J., H. Galbo, N.J. Christensen, H.-H. Parving, and J. Benn. Haemodynamic changes during graded exercise in patients with diabetic autonomic neuropathy. *Diabetologia*, 22:318-323, 1982.

26. Horvath, S.M. Review of energetics and blood flow in exercise. *Diabetes*, 28 (suppl.), 1:33-38, 1979.

27. Huttunen, N.-P., M.-L. Kärr, R. Puukka, and H.K. Akerblom. Exercise-induced proteinuria in children and adolescents with type I (insulin-dependent) diabetes. *Diabetologia*, 21:495-497, 1981.

28. Karlefors, T. Circulatory studies during exercise with particular reference to diabetics. *Acta Med. Scand.*, 180 (suppl.), 449:3-80, 1966.

29. Kernell, A. Vitreous fluorophotometry in insulin-dependent diabetes mellitus. Experimental and clinical studies. *Linköping University Medical Dissertations*, No. 129, 1982.

30. Koivisto, V.A., and P. Felig. Effects of leg exercise on insulin absorption in diabetic patients. *N. Engl. J. Med.*, 298:77-83, 1978.

31. Koivisto, V.A., V.R. Soman, R. DeFronzo, and P. Felig. Effects of acute exercise and training on insulin binding to monocytes and insulin sensitivity in vivo. *Acto Paediatr. Scand. Suppl.*, 283:70-78, 1980.

32. Larsson, Y., B. Persson, G. Sterky, and C. Thorén. Functional adaptation to rigorous training and exercise in diabetic and nondiabetic adolescents. *J. Appl. Phys.*, 19:629-635, 1964 a.

33. Larsson, Y., B. Persson, G. Sterky, and C. Thorén. Effect of exercise on blood-lipids in juvenile diabetes. *Lancet*, 1:350-355, 1964 b.

34. Larsson, Y., G. Sterky, K. Ekengren, and T. Möller. Physical fitness and the influence of training in diabetic adolescent girls. *Diabetes*, 11:109-117, 1962.

35. Lawrence, R.D. The effects of exercise on insulin action in diabetes. *Br. Med. J.*, 1:648-652, 1926.

36. Ludvigsson, J. Physical exercise in relation to degree of metabolic control in juvenile diabetics. *Acta Paediatr. Scand. Suppl.*, 283:45-49, 1980.

37. Ludvigsson, J., Y. Larsson, and P.G. Svensson. Attitudes towards physical exercise in juvenile diabetics. *Acta Paediatr. Scand. Suppl.*, 283:106-111, 1980.

38. Maehlum, S. and E.D.R. Pruett. Muscular exercise in male juvenile diabetics. II. Glucose tolerance after exercise. *Scand. J. Clin. Lab. Invest.*, 32:149-153, 1973.

39. Marble, A., P. White, R.F. Bradley, and L.P. Krall. (Eds.) *Joslin's diabetes mellitus.* 11th Ed. Philadelphia: Lea & Febiger, 1971.

40. Mogensen, C.E., and E. Vittinghus. Urinary albumin excretion during exercise in juvenile diabetes. A provocation test for early abnormalities. *Scand. J. Clin. Lab. Invest.*, 35:295, 1975.

41. Pedersen, O., H. Beck-Nielsen, and L. Heding. Increased insulin receptors after exercise in patients with insulin-independent diabetes mellitus. *N. Engl. J. Med.*, 302:886-892, 1980.

42. Persson, B., and C. Thorén. Prolonged exercise in adolescent boys with juvenile diabetes mellitus. Circulatory and metabolic responses in relation to perceived exertion. *Acta Paediatr. Scand. Suppl.*, 283:62-69, 1980.

43. Peterson, Ch.M., R.L. Jones, J.A. Esterly, G.E. Wantz, and R.L. Jackson. Changes in basement membrane thickening and pulse volume concomitant with improved glucose control and exercise in patients with insulin dependent diabetes mellitus. *Diabetes Care*, 3:586-589, 1980.

44. Pette, D., and C. Spamer. Metabolic subpopulations of muscle fibers — A quantitative study. *Diabetes*, 28 (suppl.), 1:25-29, 1979.

45. Rutenfranz, J., R. Mocellin, J. Bauer, and W. Herzig. Untersuchungen über die körperlichen Leistungsfähigkeit gesunder und kranker Heranwachsender. II. Die Leistungsfähigkeit von Kindern und Jugendlichen mit Diabetes mellitus. *Z. Kinderheilkd.*, 103:133-139, 1968.

46. Saltin, B., M. Houston, E. Nygaard, T. Graham, and J. Wahren. Muscle fiber characteristics in healthy men and patients with juvenile diabetes. *Diabetes*, 28 (suppl), 1:93-99, 1979 a.

47. Saltin, B., F. Lindgärde, M. Houston, R. Hörlin, E. Nygaard, and P. Gad. Physical training and glucose tolerance in middle-aged men with chemical diabetes. *Diabetes*, 28 (suppl.), 1:30-32, 1979 b.

48. Sterky. G. Physical work capacity in diabetic schoolchildren. *Acta Paediatr. Scand.*, 52:1-10, 1963.

49. Sterky. G., Y. Larsson, and B. Persson. Blood lipids in diabetic and nondiabetic schoolchildren. *Acta Paediatr. Scand.*, 52:11-21, 1963.

50. Sundqvist, G. Creating an interest in exercise. *Acta Paediatr. Scand. Suppl.*, 283:112-116, 1980.

51. Sundkvist, G. *Autonomic neuropathy in diabetes mellitus—With special reference to test procedures, peripheral circulation, and endothelial function.* Doctoral dissertation, Malmo, 1982.

52. Thorén, C. Exercise testing in children. *Paediatrician*, 7:100-115, 1978.

53. Vranic, M., and M. Berger. Exercise and diabetes mellitus—Review and abstracts. *Diabetes*, 28:147-163, 1979.

54. Wahren, J., P. Felig. and L. Hagenfeldt. Physical exercise and fuel homeostasis in diabetes mellitus. *Diabetologia*, 14:213-222, 1978.

55. Wallberg-Henriksson, H., R. Gunnarsson, J. Henriksson, R. De Fronzo, P. Felig, J. Östman, J. Wahren. Increased peripheral insulin sensitivity and muscle oxidative enzymes but unchanged blood glucose control in type I diabetics after physical training. *Diabetes,* 31:1044-1050, 1982.

7

The Pediatric Exercise ECG

Ian Balfour
St. Louis University Medical Center
and William B. Strong
Medical College of Georgia

Exercise stress tests have been used clinically for 2 decades to evaluate adults with heart disease, but only recently have these tests been used to evaluate children with heart disease. This chapter will present the indications for obtaining a pediatric exercise test, its components, and some of the normal and abnormal changes that may be observed, especially electrocardiographically.

EFFECTS OF EXERCISE
ON THE CARDIOVASCULAR SYSTEM

Exercise may be isometric (e.g., archery, wrestling) or dynamic (e.g., running, soccer). Isometric exercise tends to cause marked increases in systolic and diastolic blood pressure, with moderate increases in heart rate and cardiac output. Systemic vascular resistance may increase during isometric exercise. In contrast, dynamic exercise causes marked increases in heart rate and cardiac output. Systolic blood pressure will increase markedly, while diastolic blood pressure usually is unchanged but may rise or fall slightly. Systemic vascular resistance tends to fall with dynamic exercise.

Differences are also observed in left ventricular function when both types of exercise are compared. During isometric exercise left ventricular stroke volume decreases when the force of contraction is 50% or more of the maximum voluntary contraction (6). Isometric exercise is associated with an increase in end-systolic volume. Left ventricular end-diastolic volume has been found to remain unchanged during isometric exercise. In contrast, dynamic exercise results in increased stroke volume and increased shortening fraction (6), and end-systolic volume tends to decrease progressively. End-diastolic volume is thought to increase to a small degree during the initial stages of upright dynamic exercise, and then remain constant. The initial increase has been attributed to the increased venous return from exercising leg muscles. This initial rise is not seen in supine dynamic exercise.

STRESS TESTS

The exercise electrocardiogram (ECG) is usually obtained as part of a stress test which generally includes, in addition to the ECG, measurement of blood pressure, heart rate, and some parameter of work performed such as physical working capacity, oxygen consumption, or METS.

Presented below are the indications for obtaining an exercise ECG.

1. An ECG should be obtained routinely during stress tests as an aid in monitoring the subject and in providing early recognition of potentially harmful complications such as arrhythmia (3) and ischemia.

2. In patients known to have arrhythmias, stress tests can be used to either provoke the arrhythmias or to observe the response of the arrhythmia to exercise (12).

3. An ECG can detect arrhythmias in patients likely to be at increased risk of developing them (e.g., post-operative patients with tetralogy of Fallot (9), mitral prolapse).

4. An ECG can evaluate medical therapy for arrhythmias by repeating tests after initiating treatment.

5. An ECG can determine the presence or severity of lesions which may interfere with myocardial oxygen supply, such as aortic stenosis.

In isometric tests, muscle tension (contraction) is sustained against a fixed resistance such as a hand dynamometer. Because it is difficult to sustain maximum contraction for a period long enough for recordings to be made, isometric tests are usually performed at a predetermined percentage of maximum voluntary contraction, such as 30% of maximum. Dynamic tests involve alternating contraction and relaxation of opposing large muscle groups, and they may be submaximal or maximal. In submaximal tests, the subject is exercised until a predetermined amount of work has been performed or until he/she has achieved a predetermined heart rate (e.g., 85% to 90% of predicted maximum heart rate for age). In maximal tests, the subject is exercised to the point of exhaustion, which is commonly expressed as maximum voluntary effort. Dynamic tests may be further categorized into continuous and intermittent types. In both types, the subject's workload is increased at set intervals. In intermittent tests, the subject is allowed to rest before exercising against the next increase in workload. Subjects undergoing continuous tests are not allowed rest periods. Tests that increase the work load at intervals are also called graded exercise tests (GXT).

The Pediatric Performance Laboratory of the Section of Pediatric Cardiology at the Medical College of Georgia uses a continuous dynamic exercise protocol (see Figure 7-1). The child sits upright on an electronically braked cycle ergometer (Siemens 380B or a Monark mechanically braked cycle ergometer) and pedals at a constant rate. The resistance against which he or she pedals is increased at 3-minute intervals until exhaustion. Before starting the test, a full 12-lead ECG is obtained.

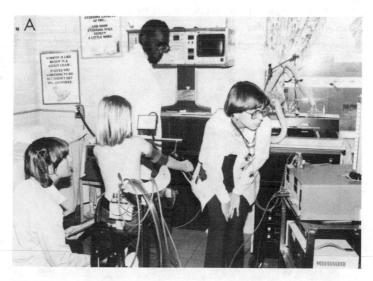

Figure 7-1. Pediatric physical performance laboratory during a cycle ergometer exercise test.

During the test, lead V5 is monitored continuously on an oscilloscope and all 12 leads are recorded during the last 10 seconds of each minute of exercise, and immediately postexercise, and at 1, 3, and 7 minutes of the postexercise recovery period. To ensure that the recordings are clear and free of artifact, the subject's skin is prepared with acetone which, apart from cleaning the skin, abraids it and decreases the amount of lipid present that can diminish electrical impedance. Silver/Silver Choloride disposable electrodes are used. The ECG is recorded using a Seimens-Elema Minograph 61. A Cambridge Electrocardiograph Model No. 3044C is used to monitor lead V5. Recently we have begun to measure blood pressure (BP) with a Critikon 1165 automatic sphygmomanometer. Previously, BP was measured manually using a mercury sphygmomanometer. Blood pressure is measured with the subject's right arm resting on an adjustable stand (Figure 7-2), which diminishes the motion of the arm and, hence, artifact.

The subject's starting workload is calculated from graphs of maximum workload plotted against body surface area (obtained from studies of normal subjects). The subject's body surface area is calculated from the Dubois nomogram. The maximum workload corresponding to the 50th percentile for the subject's BSA is found from charts of normal patients (see Figure 7-3). For example, a subject with a BSA of $1.25M^2$, the 50th percentile for maximum workload, is 600 KpM. This value is divided by 3 and the subject is started at a load of 200 KpM, the load being increased by this value at 3-minute intervals (i.e., 200 KpM at minute 1, 400 KpM at minute 4, 600 KpM at minute 7) until the subject is exhausted. A kilopond or Kp is an internationally used unit of work, and is the force acting on one kilogram at the acceleration of gravity.

The increased muscular work involved in stress tests requires an increased oxygen supply to the contracting muscles. To effect one's in-

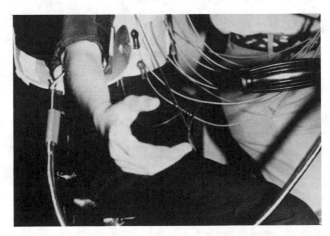

Figure 7-2. Adjustable stand supports subject's arm while blood pressure is measured.

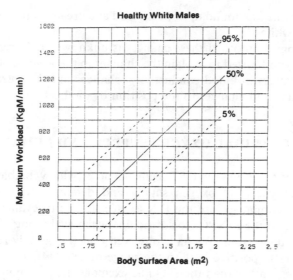

Figure 7-3. Maximum workload vs. body surface area, 5th, 50th, and 95th percentiles are shown.

crease in oxygen supply, an increase in oxygen intake and cardiac output must occur. The stress test may therefore be used in evaluating the cardiovascular, musculoskeletal, and respiratory systems separately or collectively. In children, most tests are carried out to objectively evaluate the subject's physical working capacity, myocardial oxygen supply and demand, arrhythmia detection and/or provocation, and to evaluate blood pressure response. In adult stress tests, the focus originally was on the ECG ischemic response and only more recently on arrhythmia evaluation.

Some of the changes that may occur in the exercise ECG as compared to the resting ECG include: increased amplitude of the P waves; shortening of all intervals in the R-R interval with the exception of the QRS interval; decrease in the R wave amplitude, with a shift of the QRS vector to the right; increase in the S wave amplitude, initially a decrease in the T wave amplitude with mild exercise but increased amplitude above resting values at maximum exercise.

Work performed in our pediatric performance laboratory has elicited differences in the ECGs of black children and white children (2). The resting R wave tends to be of greater amplitude in black girls when compared to their white counterparts. In both groups the R wave decreases during exercise but the same relative black-white difference persists. No significant difference was noted between black boys and white boys. Black girls also tended to have deeper S waves at rest and maximum exercise than white girls. No difference was found between blacks and whites in the degree of J point elevation at maximum exercise. Some difference in J point elevation was observed at rest and at lower levels of exercise.

The ST segment was found to slope upward at a greater rate in the blacks than in the whites.

The etiology of most of these changes is unknown. Different reasons have been hypothesized to explain the changes in the R wave (4). Among these are changes in blood conductivity, changes in left ventricular size and geometry, and changes in the position of the heart.

MYOCARDIAL OXYGEN SUPPLY AND DEMAND

Evaluation of the J point and ST segment can provide valuable information about myocardial oxygen supply and demand. At the Medical College of Georgia, we use the P-R isoelectric line to evaluate J point depression, and the PQ-PQ isoelectric line when evaluating ST segment elevation or depression. We have observed that this greatly reduces the number of false positive tests to the range of 2% (14). Using the P-R isoelectric line rather than the P-Q line excludes the possibility of atrial depolarization causing false positive readings for J point depression (see Figure 7-4). The ST segment tends to slope upward with exercise. Flattening or depression of the first 60 msec of the ST segment has been associated with the ischemia (5) in adult studies and corroborated in children using radionuclide testing (see Figure 7-5). Both the J point and ST segment have been used in assessing ischemia, since we have found this combination increases the specificity in making the diagnosis. From our studies on healthy children, we have found 2.3% to have J point depression at maximum exercise and only 1 of 170 healthy children to have ST depression with maximum exercise. However, no healthy children have had both J point and ST depression (11,14). Figure 7-6 il-

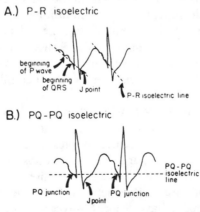

Figure 7-4. Two methods of measuring J-point. In the PR isoelectric method a line is drawn from the onset of P wave to the onset of QRS complex. This method avoids the artifact of J-point depression caused by atrial repolarization—the TA-wave. In the PQ-PQ isoelectric method, a line is drawn from the beginning of the QRS complex to the beginning of next.

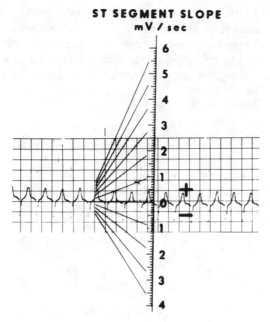

ST SEGMENT SLOPE
mV / sec

Figure 7-5. Method of measurement of ST segment. The slope of a tangent to the ST segment 60-80msec after the J-point is estimated to the nearest 0.5mV/sec.

Pediatric "Ischemic Response"

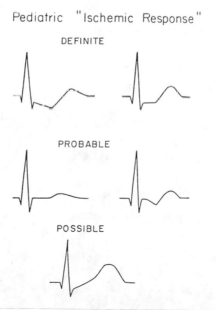

DEFINITE

PROBABLE

POSSIBLE

Figure 7-6. Patterns of ECG response in ischemia. Possible: J-point displacement with upward sloping ST segment. Probable: no displacement of J-point, but flattened or depressed ST segment. Definite: J-point displacement with flattened or downward sloping ST segment.

lustrates the gradations of ischemic changes and Figures 7 and 8 are examples of ischemic responses to exercise. Lesions commonly associated with ischemic changes are: aortic stenosis, hypertrophic obstructive cardiomyopathy, sickle cell anemia, aberrant left coronary artery, and mitral prolapse, the latter for reasons yet to be determined.

Resting HR 88

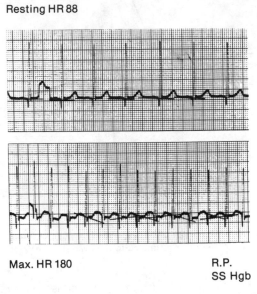

Max. HR 180   R.P.
                                     SS Hgb

Figure 7-7. J-point displacement and flat ST segment at maximum exercise in a patient with sickle cell anemia.

Stage II   Minute 6   HR$_1$ 182   P.T.-092-165

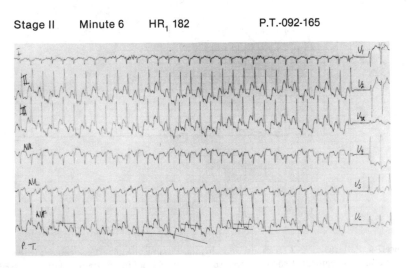

Figure 7-8. J-point displacement and inverted T-wave in a patient with mitral valve prolapse.

ARRHYTHMIAS

Stress tests may provoke, alter, or abolish conduction defects and arrhythmias (7,8). The stress test is also thought to provide a greater yield than Holter monitoring in the detection of arrhythmias (10,11).

Exercise causes an increase in sympathetic activity and a decrease in vagal activity. These changes in the autonomic nervous system result in an increase in the rate of depolarization of the myocardial cells (7,9,12) and may result in possible foci of arrhythmias discharging. This is especially likely if there are areas of myocardial injury or ischemia (8).

Benign, short-lived supraventricular arrhythmias such as wandering atrial pacemaker and atrial ectopic beats are frequently seen during the recovery period of exercise tests (7,8). Figure 7-9 demonstrates the resting and exercise study of an 8-year-old boy with a history of palpitations. He was subsequently treated with digoxin and a repeat exercise test did not provoke any arrhythmia. Some doubt has been cast on the ability of the stress test to provoke arrhythmias in patients with Wolff-Parkinson-White (WPW) or preexcitation syndrome (13). It should also be noted that the S-T depression occurring with preexcitation elicited during the test is not a reliable index of ischemia (13). Normalization of conduction has been reported to occur in WPW patients during exercise and these patients may no longer have the characteristic delta wave with a wide QRS. This change in the conduction has been theorized as being a result of increased sympathetic discharge causing conduction through the normal pathway to be faster than through the accessory pathway. Brief runs of paroxysmal atrial tachycardia and A-V junctional tachyarrhythmia have been reported as being common and benign findings in adults in the early stages of exercise. These *have not been* noted in healthy children.

Accelerated A-V conduction is expected as a normal finding as a result of increased sympathetic activity (7). Lengthening of the P-R interval is

T.L. 092-714
26 May 76

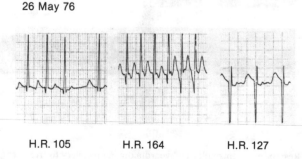

H.R. 105   H.R. 164   H.R. 127

Figure 7-9. This patient developed supraventricular tachycardia at maximum exercise.

therefore abnormal, and may be elicited along with other disturbances in conduction (e.g., A-V block, bundle branch block), during a stress test (8). A preexisting A-V block may decrease in severity during the test.

Ventricular premature beats (PVCs) are the most commonly occurring arrhythmia, and the most worrisome in view of the possibility of them inducing ventricular tachycardia/fibrillation and sudden death. PVCs are a common finding in otherwise healthy individuals and usually are present at rest and disappear with low level exercise as a result of increased

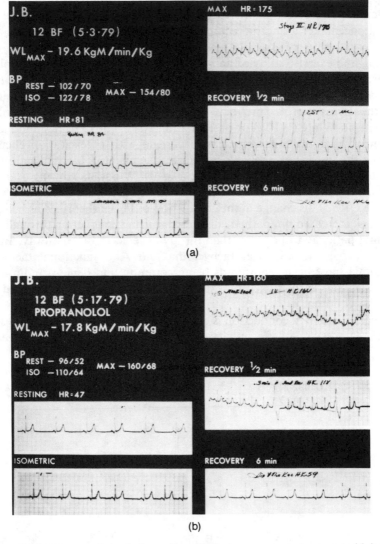

(a)

(b)

Figure 7-10. Response of ventricular tachycardia during recovery to treatment with inderal is shown.

S-A node discharge and overdrive suppression. PVCs which become more frequent as the patient's heart rate increases or which progress to ventricular tachycardia should be treated when symptomatic (1) (see Figure 7-10). However, when asymptomatic there remains some controversy as to whether or not they should be treated pharmacologically.

The following are criteria for regarding PVCs as benign: (a) unifocal; (b) not associated with underlying cardiac pathology; (c) disappear with exercise at heart rates of 150/min, that is, respond to overdrive suppression by the sinus node; (d) do not occur in the vulnerable period of repolarization; and (e) do not initiate a severe dysrhythmia (12).

CONTRAINDICATIONS TO EXERCISE TESTS

Table 7-1 lists contraindications to stress testing and medical conditions which require that special precautions be taken during the test. To these must be added the following indications for aborting the test: (a) serious dysrhythmias such as multifocal PVCs, ventricular tachycardia, supraventricular tachycardia, or high degree of A-V block; (b) potential hazards to the patients such as failure of monitoring equipment, dizziness, or syncope precipitated by exercise; and inappropriate rise or fall in systolic and diastolic blood pressure.

Although this presentation has dealt with the exercise ECG, one should not forget that the patient's history and physical examination are equally important. The history may reveal a high intake of stimulants (e.g., caffeine, cola, tea). Symptoms such as fainting, dizziness, chest pain or easy fatigability are equally important in deciding on a plan for a patient. Physical examination may reveal abnormalities such as mitral valve prolapse or evidence of left ventricular outflow obstruction. Exercise testing is used to assess the functional capabilities and responses of the cardiovascular system. It is not generally a diagnostic test except when dysrhythmia may be provoked.

Table 7-1

Contraindications for Exercise Stress Testing

Acute illness
    Cardiac (i.e., myocarditis, pericarditis, angina at rest, and myocardial infarction)
    Noncardiac—febrile illnesses, respiratory illness (e.g., acute asthma, thrombophlebitis)

Uncontrolled active chronic systemic disease
    Cardiac—congestive heart failure
    Noncardiac—thyroid, renal, hepatic

Table 7-2

**Conditions Requiring Special Care
During Exercise Stress Testing***

Moderate or severe aortic stenosis
Marked cardiomegaly
Severe pulmonary hypertension
Poorly controlled systemic hypertension
Conduction disturbances—second- or third-degree AV block, pacemakers,
   trifascicular block
Uncontrolled dysrhythmias
Hypoxemia
Severe anemia or polycythemia

*From the Exercise Committee of the American Heart Association.

By means of the stress test and stress ECG, the adolescent with nonspecific chest pain can be objectively evaluated and, when found to have a normal test, can be reassured and encouraged to be normally active. This often provides all the assurance the family and child needs to be normally active.

SUMMARY

This has been a brief review of pediatric stress testing, especially the exercise ECG. The child with cardiac, respiratory, or other diseases can be evaluated in order to objectively determine his or her exercise capability so that he or she will not be unduly restricted, but appropriate restrictions may be instituted if needed.

REFERENCES

1. Alpert, B.S., J. Boineau, and W.B. Strong. Exercise induced ventricular tachycardia. *Ped. Cardiol.,* 2:51-55, 1982.

2. Alpert, B.S., N.L. Flood, W.B. Strong, B. Dover, R. Du Rant, A.M. Martin, and D.L. Booker. Responses to ergometer exercise in a healthy biracial population of children. *J. Pediatr.* (In press).

3. Antman, A., T.B. Graboys, and B. Lown. Continuous monitoring for ventricular arrhythmias during exercise test. *JAMA,* 241:2802-2805, 1979.

4. Baron, D.W., C. Ilsley, I. Sheiban, P.A. Poole-Wilson, and A.F. Richards. R wave amplitude during exercise. Relation to left ventricular function and coronary artery disease. *Brit. Heart J.,* 44:512-517, 1980.

5. Chahine, R.A., M.R. Awdeh, M. Mnayer, A.E. Raizner, and R.J. Luchi. The evolutionary pattern of exercise-induced ST segment depression. *J. Electrocard.,* 12(3):235-239, 1979.

6. Crawford, M.H., D.H. White, and K.W. Amon. Echocardiographic evaluation of left ventricular size and performance during handgrip and supine and upright bicycle exercise. *Circulation,* 59:1188-1196, 1979.

7. DeMaria, A.N., Z. Vera, E.A. Amsterdam, D.T. Mason, and R.A. Massumi. Disturbances of cardiac rhythm and conduction induced by exercise. *Amer. J. Cardiol.,* 33:732-736, 1974.

8. Goldberg, A.N. Exercise stress testing in uncovering of dysrhythmias. *Med. Clinics of N.A.,* 60(2), 1976.

9. Goldschlager, N., K. Cohn, and A. Goldschlager. Exercise related ventricular arrhythmias. *Mod. Concepts of Cardiovasc. Dis.,* 47(12):67-72, 1979.

10. Graboys, T.B., and R.F. Wright. Provocation of supraventricular tachycardia during exercise stress testing. *Cardiovasc. Reviews and Reports,* 1(1):57-58, 1980.

11. Kulangara, R.J., and W.B. Strong. Exercise stress testing in children. *Comprehensive Therapy,* 5(6), 1979.

12. Monarrez, C.N., W.B. Strong, and A.H. Rees. Exercise electrocardiography in the evaluation of cardiac dysrhythmias in children. *Paediatrician,* 7:116-125, 1978.

13. Strasberg, B., W.W. Ashley, C.R.C. Wyndham, R.A. Bauernfeind, S.P. Swiryn, R.C. Dhingra, and K.M. Rosen. Treadmill exercise testing in the Wolff-Parkinson-White syndrome. *Amer. J. Cardiol.,* 45:742-747, 1980.

14. Thapar, M.K., W.B. Strong, M.D. Miller, L. Leatherbury, and M. Salebhai. Exercise electrocardiography of healthy black children *Amer. J. Dis. Child.,* 132:592-595, 1978.

8

Coronary Heart Disease Risk in Children and Their Physical Activity Patterns

Thomas B. Gilliam
TBG Enterprises, Inc., Twinsburg, Ohio
and Susan E. MacConnie
University of Michigan

Coronary heart disease (CHD) risk factors such as hypertension, obesity, elevated blood lipids, diabetes, and physical inactivity are common in children. For example, Lauer et al. (20) noted 24% of the 5,000 children examined had total cholesterol (TC) levels > 220 mg/dl, 20% were > 110% relative body weight, and after the age of 9, 19% had diastolic blood pressures > 94 mg Hg. These findings are similar to those reported by Wilmore and McNamara (38) and Gilliam et al. (10).

Since no longitudinal studies have examined the question of whether early childhood control of CHD risk factors will reduce the risk of fatal heart attack or the incidence of heart disease (and whether the reverse is true) in adult life, policies, procedures, and recommendations depend on circumstantial evidence from a variety of sources. However, there is little doubt concerning the association of risk factors in adults and the incidence of CHD. Epidemiological studies have provided such evidence. The Pooling Project of the U.S. (26) which combined data from five areas of the country demonstrated the increased risk of CHD with increases in the levels of TC (> 240 = 2 × risk of someone < 218 mg/dl), systolic and diastolic pressure (> 177 mm Hg, SBP ≈ 3.5 × risk of someone at 120; > 94 mm Hg DBP = 2.2 × risk), smoking (1 + pk/day = 2.5 × risk, > 1 + pk/day = 3.2 × risk) and obesity (mostly related to 40- to 45-year-olds and more associated with presence of other risk factors). The concern with obesity is more related to its association with primary risk factors such as hypertension and hypercholesterolemia.

These data are supported by results from autopsies and animal studies. The International Atherosclerosis Project (IAP) as reported by McGill et al. (22) demonstrated that the extent of atherosclerotic lesions, in carefully controlled analyses, were related to total cholesterol, dietary saturated and total fat, and smoking habits. In addition, many animal studies such as those done by Wissler (39), Kramsch et al. (18), and Ross and Harker (28) have demonstrated greater numbers and more extensive lesions in hypercholesterolemic animals. Kramsch et al. (18) demonstrated significantly more EKG abnormalities in monkeys with high TC levels.

The explanation of how this data relates to a child with elevated risk factors requires a synthesis of data from several areas. First, one must consider the natural progression of the atherosclerotic plaque, and whether it is a phenomenon of aging. Evidence from autopsy data suggests the atherosclerotic process begins in childhood. Strong and McGill (22,32,33) have reported data from the IAP that demonstrate the presence of fatty streaks in the aortas of some children < 3 years of age, and in all children examined > 3 years. The presence of fatty streaks in the coronary artery is delayed somewhat, but they were present in some children < 10 years, with increasing number > 10 years and in all subjects > 20 years of age. Velican and Velican (40,41) also noted changes in the intima that could be associated with plaque formation between the ages of 5-10 years with a "critical period" observed between age or groups of 11-15 and 16-20 years, noting a large increase in the presence of lesions.

These data, plus the data of Enos et al. (8) and McNamara et al. (23) — who respectively noted that 77% of Korean casualties and 46% of the Vietnam casualties had atherosclerotic lesions with varying degrees of severity — provide evidence of the early beginnings of atherosclerosis. Concerning the fatty streak, there is evidence for and against its role as a precursor for plaque formation. Evidence by Pearson et al. (25), who noted two types of fatty streaks with one type similar to the monoclonal type observed by Benditt and Benditt (1), suggests that some of the fatty streaks might be precursors. This evidence supports the notion that the atherosclerotic process begins early in life.

The idea that atherogenesis begins in early life has provided the impetus to screen young children for CHD risk and note the course of these levels through young adulthood. As stated earlier, the prevalence of risk factors in children has been reported by many investigators. Lauer et al. (20) reporting data from the Muscatine (Iowa) prevalence study noted that 24% of the approximately 5,000 children (8-16 yrs.) had TC > 200 md/dl, 9% > 220 and 1% > 240 mg/dl, 9% had systolic blood pressures (SPB) > 140 mm, 12% had diastolic blood pressures (DBP) > 90 mm HG, and 20-25% had relative weights > 110%. Wilmore and McNamara (38) and Gilliam et al. (10) also noted that > 50% of the children tested had one or more risk factors (elevated blood pressure, elevated TC, elevated triglycerides, or elevated body fat). Perhaps more important is the clustering of risk factors noted by Khoury et al. (16). This group observed that children classified as at high risk, by virtue of their high low-density lipoprotein cholesterol (LDL-C) levels and low high-density lipoprotein cholesterol (HDL-C) levels, also had the highest quetelet index, the highest skinfold measurements, and above average SBP. This would substantially increase their risk if these were maintained into adulthood.

Childhood risk factors might not be of concern if the child outgrew those elevated levels. Several investigators have examined the phenomenon of "tracking" in children. Although this has been done on a small scale (approximately 100 children), the data do provide some insight into this important area. Laskarzewski et al. (19) examined blood lipids of children classified in the 95th percentile for TC, LDL-C, Triglyceride (TG), and HDL-C. He noted that while dispersion occurred over a 4-year period (11-15 yrs. of age), there was a significant tendency for these levels to remain high. TC, TG, and HDL maintained a high frequency in the 95th percentile. While a few children decreased their values, the mode remained at the 95th percentile. LDL-C showed more dispersion with the mode slipping to the 90th percentile. However, most of the children whose LDL-C decreased remained in the upper 30%. In all of the parameters there was a correlation between the decrease values and the expected decrease due to regression toward the means. Fredrichs et al., as reported by Voller and Strong (42) in 1981, have also observed tracking for blood pressure and obesity in children. Thus it appears that although more needs to be done in this area, preliminary evidence shows that children with high levels of blood pressure, lipids, and obesity tend to retain those high levels, and this could increase their adult risk.

Special population groups provide further information on what levels might be desirable especially for blood lipids. The multifactorial nature of atherosclerosis makes complete determination difficult, but some information can be gleaned from these groups. Data reported by Goldstein and Brown (13,14) on genetic lipid metabolism disorders supports the importance of lipid levels. Heterzygotes for familial hypercholesterolemia develop CHD complication by the age of 30 with substantially elevated LDL-C levels. Homozygotes have cholesterol levels > 400 mg/dl and usually develop clinical symptoms before the age of 20. At the other extreme are populations known to have low CHD incidence. Strong and McGill (22,32,33) noted that in those countries, lesion number and extent, as well as progression, is lower than in high CHD-incidence countries. Total cholesterol levels in such groups generally fall between 120-140 mg/dl, as reported by Blackburn (2). Furthermore, populations in which CHD incidence is low, and both children and adults have been measured, show both groups having lower lipids than populations in high CHD areas. For example, Savage et al. (30) reported that in the Pima Indians, a group with low CHD incidence, the TC levels of the children were 125 mg/dl and the adults level was maintained at an average of 190 mg/dl. This was compared to Tecumseh, Michigan, in which the TC levels increased to approximately 220 mg/dl with increased age (30). The Tarahumara Indians also have lower CHD and lower blood lipids both in children and adults (118 mg/dl and 125 mg/dl respectively) (4).

The evidence cited above suggests that the typical increase built into standards for risk factors due to aging may not be justified. Marmot (24) recently stated that "the epidemiological evidence suggests that the rate of occurrence of CHD is largely determined by the environment" (p. 332). It follows that intervention programs early in life may help prevent CHD.

Physical activity and weight control have been suggested as forms of early intervention because many studies show that increased levels of physical activity and ideal body weight maintenance reduce CHD risks in adults. Those intervention programs have been specifically reported to decrease fat weight, increase high-density lipoprotein cholesterol, decrease triglyceride values, increase maximal oxygen consumption, reduce resting heart rate, reduce systolic blood pressure, and lower blood glucose levels.

CHILDHOOD OBESITY

Environmental factors such as overeating and physical inactivity have been identified as leading causes of childhood obesity. Several studies have reported that obese boys do not necessarily eat more than their nonobese peers. For example, Johnson et al. (15) showed that obese high school girls consumed 8225.49 kJ daily in comparison to 11327.32 kJ for control girls. Both groups were classified as sedentary although the control girls were significantly more active in sports and other strenuous activities as determined through interviews. Similar findings were reported by Rose and Mayer (27) for infants. That is, obese infants tended to be hypoactive and consume fewer calories than their nonobese counterparts. In contrast, Waxman and Stunkard (36) reported that obese boys expend more energy and consume more calories than nonobese boys. However, since body weight influences energy expenditure, it is more meaningful to express energy expenditure relative to body weight. When correcting their data for body weight, the energy expenditure and intake for these obese boys was either equal to or less than for the nonobese boys. Recently Saris et al. (29) reported that less active children (ages 4 to 6) consumed fewer calories when compared to more active children, with no differences observed in body weight and skinfold measures. However, with older children (ages 8 to 12), the less active ones tended to weigh more and have more body fat but consume the same number of calories as the more active group of children.

In a recent pilot project using Holter devices to monitor physical activity patterns in obese ($n = 5$) and nonobese ($n = 5$) boys, Gilliam showed that obese boys do not expend as many calories per unit body weight as lean boys and may even consume fewer calories (Tables 8-1 and 8-2). However, the obese boys were just as active as the lean boys when

Table 8-1

Physical Characteristics, and Blood Lipid and Lipoproteins of Lean ($n = 5$) and Obese ($n = 5$) Boys

Variables	Lean M	S.D.	Obese M	S.D.	†-Statistic
Age (months)	84.0 ±	2.55	85.2 ±	5.26	0.46
Weight (kg)	21.4 ±	1.61	28.9 ±	2.72	5.34[a]
Height (cm)	115.9 ±	4.14	124.9 ±	2.39	4.20[a]
Quetelet index (x1000)	1.6 ±	0.07	1.85 ±	0.11	4.52[a]
Sum of skinfolds (mm)	19.8 ±	1.72	44.7 ±	17.48	3.18[a]
Resting heart rate (bpm^{-1})	86 ±	9.8	88 ±	3.30	0.39
Cholesterol (mg/dl)	154.4 ±	23.60	161.2 ±	31.67	0.38
LDL-cholesterol (mg/dl)	90.4 ±	11.85	98.2 ±	24.96	0.63
HDL-cholesterol (mg/dl)	47.0 ±	5.70	44.8 ±	14.31	0.32
Triglycerides (mg/dl)	44.2 ±	12.66	50.0 ±	28.85	0.42
VLDL-Triglycerides (mg/dl)	16.8 ±	10.00	20.6 ±	19.41	0.39
HDL/LDL (X100)	52.4 ±	6.57	45.5 ±	6.54	1.68

[a]$t_{8df} = 2.31, p \leq 0.05$

Table 8-2

Energy Intake and Expenditure
for Lean ($n = 5$) and Obese ($n = 5$) Boys

Variable	Lean M	Lean S.D.	Obese M	Obese S.D.	t-Statistic
Energy intake (kJ)	8007.8	± 2575.69	8426.4	± 1973.11	0.29
Energy expended (kJ)	7472.0	± 1007.53	7894.8	± 1940.4	0.43
Energy intake kJ•kg^{-1})	372.1	± 112.65	296.0	± 84.98	1.20
Energy expended (kJ•ml•kg^{-1})	0.486 ±	0.0536	0.377 ±	0.0762	2.61[a]

[a] $t_{8df} = 2.31, p < 0.05$

comparing their physical activity profile. Both groups of boys were involved in high intensity activity (i.e., HR > 150 bpm^{-1}) for about the same duration (Table 8-3). Minute-by-minute heart rates grouped into 10-bpm categories showed the total time the heart beat was within each category for the lean and the obese boys. Even though statistically no differences between the two groups for the heart rate category 120-149 bpm^{-1} were obtained, a larger sample size might have lent greater significance since absolute differences were so great in favor of the obese boys. That is, during the 12-hour period (720 minutes) the cumulative total time the obese boys' heart rate fell within this category was 154.4 minutes in comparison to 81.7 minutes for the lean boys. This reflects a greater involvement in moderate intensity activity for the obese boys.

Statistically, no differences between the groups for any of the blood lipids were obtained, but there is a trend which indicates lower LDL-C and TG and higher HDL-C for the leaner boys. Similar findings have been reported for adults and children. For example, a tendency toward lower HDL-C values and higher cholesterol and LDL-C values was reported by Weninger et al. (37), for 10 grossly obese children compared to 64 normal weight children.

Table 8-3

Group	Heart Rate Categories (bpm^{-1}) 80-89	90-99	100-109	110-119	120-129
Lean	95.6	223.7	199.7	90.1	42.1
Obese	104.9	128.1	171.8	129.2	86.1

The importance of controlling obesity in early childhood is related to its association with other CHD risk factors, primarily lipid and carbohydrate metabolism. Excess caloric intake is associated with increased cholesterol synthesis by the liver and thus increased serum cholesterol levels. Perhaps more important is the association with hyperinsulinemia due to decreased receptor sensitivity to insulin. The result of this insensitivity is increased production of FFA and therefore an increased synthesis of triglycerides. Since very low density lipoprotein (VLDL) is synthesized in relation to the amount of TG to be transported, an increased VLDL secretion is observed (6). This would not present a problem if catabolism increased, but Taskinen and Nikkila (34) reported that in obesity, lipoprotein lipase (LPL) is also less sensitive, thereby decreasing VLDL catabolism. Exercise would not only increase energy expenditure and maintain caloric balance but also increase the sensitivity of the receptors to insulin. Terjung (35) noted that in obese subjects who exercise, even without losing weight, insulin sensitivity would improve and this would help reduce the effect of hyperinsulinemia. In addition, the increase in LPL noted with training would improve the catabolism of VLDL that was produced.

The composition of diet is critical in controlling body weight of children. Unfortunately, the pediatric diet cannot be addressed at this time other than to acknowledge the *importance* of integrating physical activity and dietary intervention programs in dealing with obesity and associated disorders.

PHYSICAL ACTIVITY

As stated earlier, adult studies show that increased levels of physical activity reduce coronary heart disease risks. However, there has been some question as to whether or not the benefits derived from exercise normally observed in adults will occur in children. Several studies have revealed that trained prepubescent children do not differ physiologically from their untrained counterparts. Apparently a maturational threshold exists whereby prepubescent children are unable to elicit physiological changes in response to exercise training. For example, several studies (5,7,9,17)

Minute-by-Minute Heart Rates Grouped into 10-bpm^{-1} Categories

		Heart Rate Categories (bpm^{-1})			
130-139	140-149	150-159	160-169	170-179	>180
22.7	16.9	11.1	8.2	4.2	5.9
42.9	25.4	13.2	6.3	6.3	5.7

have reported no differences in aerobic power between prepubescent control and experimental children. However, those studies show significantly higher aerobic power values in experimental postpubescent children.

Why is it, then, that young children (i.e., prepubescent children) do not show increases in aerobic power as a result of physical training programs? Could it be because they are naturally more active at this age than they are in the postpubescent stages?

At present little is known about physical activity patterns of children. That is, do children experience vigorous physical activity (heart rate 160 bpm^{-1}) on a regular basis? If not, can their activity patterns be modified to include more intense activity in their daily routine? It has been suggested that the physical activity sessions for adults should consist of 25-30 minutes of continuous exercise at an intensity sufficient to elicit a target heart rate of at least 60% of the individual's heart rate range (HR max − HR rest). Applied to children, these adult standards would yield a target heart rate of at least 160 bpm^{-1}.

Gilliam et al. (11) reported that voluntary activity patterns (as determined by Holter monitors) of children may be inadequate in terms of duration and intensity to promote cardiovascular health. That is, in a 12-hour ($n = 720$ min) monitoring period during the summer, 7-year-old boys and girls achieved heart rates greater than 159 bpm^{-1} for only 21 and 9 minutes, respectively. Saris et al. (29) recorded heart rate data for 24 hours during the school year on 171 kindergarteners, ages 4 to 6, and 54 elementary school children, ages 8 to 12, who were divided into low and high activity groups. The length of time kindergarten children had heart rates greater than 176 bpm was only 15 minutes and 4 minutes for the active and less active groups, respectively, compared to 6 minutes and 4 minutes for the active and less active 8- to 12-year-old children. Seliger et al. (31), reporting 24-hour minute-by-minute heart rate data recorded during the school year on 11- and 12-year-old boys, showed that 3% of the time was spent in activities classified as moderate and medium. At no time did the boys engage in heavy intensity activity. Mean heart rates ranging from 102 to 145 bpm^{-1} were recorded by Bradfield et al. (3) during lunch and recess of 54 7- to 10-year-old boys. Frequency distributions revealed that at no time were heart rates in excess of 155 bpm^{-1}, approximately 4 minutes at heart rates of 140-155 bpm^{-1}, and 50 minutes at heart rates of 110-140 bpm^{-1} during the school day.

Recently Gilliam et al. (12) and MacConnie et al. (21) completed a physical activity intervention program designed to increase activity patterns in young children. The purpose of the exercise program was to stimulate the cardiovascular and muscular systems to enhance strength, aerobic and anaerobic capacity, flexibility, and agility. Activity patterns of children were determined during the summer before the physical activity intervention program began; then activity patterns during the school year were monitored when the physical activity intervention program was introduced.

The two school systems involved were similar in socioeconomic status and in population. One school system served as the control group in which the children participated in their traditional physical education classes. The other school system served as the experimental group in which the children participated in a high-intensity physical activity program 4 days per week, 25 minutes per session. The physical activity intervention program was designed to increase the heart rates up to and sustain them at 150 beats per minute for a 20- to 25-minute period. Physical activity patterns were monitored with a Holter device for the physical activity intervention class and the control physical education class, for a 12-hour period. The Exersentry device was also used to monitor heart rates in order to elicit immediate feedback for the children and the instructor.

Before reporting the results of the physical activity intervention program on activity patterns of these children, it is important to identify what is meant by heart rate intensities. The four heart rate categories used to identify the intensity at which the heart is beating are shown in Figure 8-1. The intensity is related to the level of physical activity. As can be observed, there are four heart rate categories: less than 121 bpm, reflecting a low activity level; 121 to 140 bpm, indicating a low/moderate activity level; 141 to 160 bpm, indicating a high/moderate activity level; and greater than 160 bpm, indicating a high level of physical activity.

What then would be the recommended heart rate intensities for a 12-hour day for a child? This can be observed in Figure 8-2. As indicated, it is recommended that a child experience 30 minutes per day in high intensity physical activities, 6% in high/moderate activities, 13% (90 minutes) in low/moderate activities, and the rest of the day, 77%, at low activity levels. These recommendations are based on the need to experience high intensity activity for 25 to 30 minutes in order to improve and maintain cardiovascular health.

Figure 8-3 shows the breakdown of the typical heart rate intensities during the summer months for girls and boys. As can be observed, the children spent 2% of their time in the high heart rate category in comparison to the recommended 4%. The children also spent 4% in the

Heart Rate Categories: Activity Level

- Less than 121 beats per minute   = Low (L)
- 121-140 beats per minute   = Low Moderate (LM)
- 141-160 beats per minute   = High Moderate (HM)
- Greater than 160 beats per minute = High (H)

Figure 8-1. Heart rate categories used during the study.

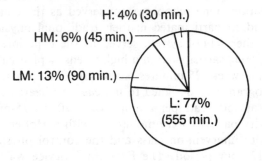

Figure 8-2. Recommended daily heart rate intensities children should experience as part of a physical activity intervention program designed to reduce CHD risk.

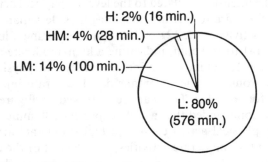

Figure 8-3. Typical heart rate intensities recorded via a Holter monitor during the summer on children ages 6-8.

high/moderate category, in comparison to the 6% that is recommended. In the low/moderate category, 14% was recommended. Also observed was that the children spent 13% of their time in the low/moderate category. The children spent 80% of their time within the low category relative to the 77% that is recommended. When the typical heart rate intensities for boys and girls were assessed independently, differences between the activity patterns of boys and girls becomes evident (Figure 8-4). In comparing the two pie graphs, it is obvious that the boys spent more time than the girls in the higher heart rate categories—greater than 141 beats per minute. Of the boys' time, a total of 56 minutes, or 8%, was spent in the two high categories, compared to 29 minutes, or only 4%, of the girls' time. Likewise, one can observe that the girls spent considerably more time in the low heart rate category than the boys. Keep in

Heart Rate Intensities During the Summer

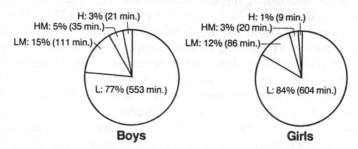

Figure 8-4. Typical heart rate intensities recorded via a Holter monitor by sex during the summer on children ages 6-8.

mind that these data reflect activity patterns prior to the physical activity intervention program. These data were collected during the summer, when the children were not restricted in any way to classroom activities.

Figure 8-5 shows the results of the intervention program. The top portion of the figure reflects the activity patterns for the control and experimental children for the high, high/moderate, low/moderate, and low categories. The bottom half of the figure shows the activity patterns for the same heart rate categories during the intervention program. As can be observed, there were no differences between the control and experimental children prior to intervention. That is, they both spent approximately 2% of their time in the high heart rate categories and 4% in the high/moderate heart rate categories. There are slight differences with the low/moderate and low categories. However, these differences were

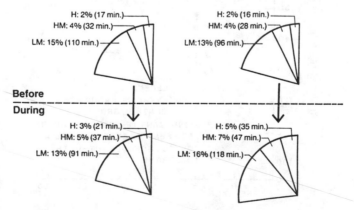

Figure 8-5. Results of heart rate intensities recorded via a Holter monitor following the physical activity intervention program on children ages 6-8.

insignificant. As a result of the intervention program, the experimental children increased their high intensity heart rate level from 16 to 35 minutes per day and the high/moderate category from 28 to 47 minutes per day, in comparison to the slight increase observed in the control children that occurred during school as opposed to their preintervention data. For the control children, the increase went from 17 minutes to 21 minutes for the high heart rate category and from 32 minutes to 37 minutes for the high/moderate heart rate category. The low/moderate and low categories did not change substantially.

Figure 8-6 shows the results of Exersentry data recorded during the physical activity intervention program and illustrates that the objective of the intervention exercise session was achieved. The mean rate for the experimental groups during the 25-minute period was 156 bpm in comparison to mean heart rate for the control group of 136 bpm. The statistical analyses revealed no significant differences between the two groups' preexercise heart rates but the experimental children had significantly ($p < .05$) higher exercise heart rates than the control children.

The results of the intervention program show that the children were more active than the physical activity intervention program itself can account for. That is, the children became more active during their voluntary time, recess, and after school. For example, the increase in time at the high and high/moderate categories was 38 minutes in comparison to the 25-minute exercise session. This also carried through to the summer months following the intervention program (unpublished results). That

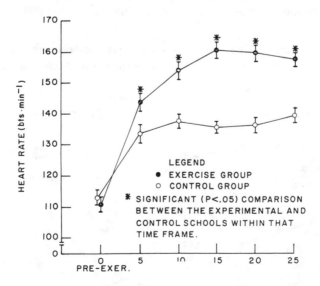

Figure 8-6. Results of heart rate (bpm^{-1}) recorded during the physical activity intervention program and controlled physical education class.

is, the experimental children were significantly more active than the control children.

As indicated earlier, gender differences were observed in the children's activity patterns. It appears from an earlier report that these gender differences can be minimized if girls are given the opportunity to participate in vigorous physical activity (12). That is, girls in the control group expended a similar amount of energy during the summer and the school year. However, girls in the experimental group showed a substantial increase in energy expenditure as a result of the physical activity intervention program. That is, girls in the low, moderate, and high activity categories increased their daily energy expenditure by 12, 21, and 33%, respectively. The increase by the girls' high category group compare favorably with the energy expenditures reported for the boys' experimental low and moderate categories.

In addition to the above heart rate activity pattern, data are reported by Gilliam et al. (10,11) and MacConnie et al. (21) in which Holter monitoring was conducted on second, fifth, and seventh graders as part of another physical activity intervention project. These data showed that activity patterns were substantially improved for the second grade children and moderately improved for the fifth graders. No changes occurred in activity habits for seventh grade boys and girls. These results, along with the data reported above, suggest the importance of early intervention programs before attitudes and habits about exercise become a barrier to enhancing exercise patterns in children.

SUMMARY

It is evident from these data that children do not participate in a significant amount of regular vigorous physical activity but that it is possible to improve their physical activity profiles if intervention programs are initiated early in life (i.e., first and second grades). We feel this is an extremely important finding which contradicts what most individuals assume — that children are naturally active. Therefore, programs and research efforts should be designed to study the long-range effect of physical activity and dietary intervention programs on CHD risk in children.

We stated in our opening remarks that no longitudinal studies have examined whether early childhood control of CHD risk factors will reduce the risk of fatal heart attack or the incidence of heart disease in adult life. Therefore, policies, procedures, and recommendations depend on circumstantial evidence from various sources. We believe the research cited above strongly advocates early CHD screening programs for children, as well as intervention programs, to maintain ideal body weight and to encourage vigorous physical activity. Whether these programs reduce the CHD risk of children as they become adults can only be answered with longitudinal studies.

The types of screening and intervention programs suggested by the current research cannot be implemented by the medical profession alone. Rather these programs, to be successful, must come from a commitment by an entire community and include a cognitive component. The physical activity intervention program should be of sufficient intensity to elevate heart rates to at least 150 bpm^{-1} for a 20- to 25-minute period. The cognitive component is critical to ensure that children understand the whys of good nutrition and of vigorous activity. This will result in behavioral changes, which will lead to voluntary decisions by children to take control of their health at an early age.

REFERENCES

1. Benditt, E.P., and J.M. Benditt. Evidence for monoclonal origins of human artherosclerotic plaque. *Proc. Nat. Acad. Sci.,* 70(6): 1753-1756, 1973.

2. Blackburn, H. Conference on the health effects of blood lipids: Optimal distributions for populations: Epidemiological section. *Prev. Med.,* 8:612-758, 1979.

3. Bradfield, R.B., H. Chan, and N.E. Bradfield. Energy expenditures and heart rates of Cambridge boys at school. *Am. J. Clin. Nutr.,* 24:1461-1466, 1971.

4. Connor, W.E., M.R. Cerqueira, M.S. Rodney, R.W. Connor, R.B. Wallace, M.R. Malinow, and H.R. Casdorph. The plasma lipid, lipoproteins, and diet of the Tarahumara Indians of Mexico. *Am. J. Clin. Nutr.,* 31:1131-1142, 1978.

5. Dobeln, W., and B.O. Ericksson. Physical training, maximal oxygen uptake and dimensions of the oxygen transporting and metabolizing organs in boys 11 to 13 years of age. *Acta. Paediatr. Scand.,* 61:653-660, 1972.

6. Eisenberg, S., and R.I. Levy. Lipoprotein metabolism. *Advn. of Lipid Res.,* 13:1-89, 1975.

7. Ekbolm, B. Effect of physical training on adolescent boys. *J. Appl. Physiol.,* 27:350-355, 1969.

8. Enos, M.J., R.H. Holmes, and J. Beyer. Coronary artery disease among United States soldiers killed in action in Korea. *JAMA,* 152(12):1090-1093, 1953.

9. Eriksson, B.O., B. Pearson, and J. Thorell. The effects of repeated prolonged exercise on plasma growth hormone, insulin, glucose, free fatty acids, glycerol lactate, and B-hydroxybutyric acid in 13-year-old boys and in adults. *Acta. Paediatr. Scand.* (suppl), 217:142-146, 1972.

10. Gilliam, T.B., V.L. Katch, W.G. Thorland, and A.W. Weltman. Prevalence of coronary heart disease risk factors in active children, 7 to 12 years of age. *Med. Sci. Sports,* 9(1):21-25, 1977.

11. Gilliam, T.B., P.S. Freedson, D.L. Geenen, and B. Shahraray. Physical activity patterns determined by heart rate monitoring in 6- to 7-year-old children. *Med. Sci. Sports Exer.,* 13(1):65-67, 1981.

12. Gilliam, T.B., S.E. MacConnie, D.L. Geenen, A.E. Pels, and P.S. Freedson. Exercise programs for children: A way to prevent heart disease. *Phys. and Sportsmed.,* 10(9):96-108, 1982.

13. Goldstein, J.L., and M.S. Brown. "Insights into the pathogenesis of atherosclerosis derived from studies of familial hypercholesterolemia." In *Metabolic risk factors in ischemic cardiovascular disease,* edited by L.A. Carlson and B. Pernow, pp. 17-34. New York: Raven Press, 1982.

14. Goldstein, J.L., and M.S. Brown. The low-density lipoprotein pathway and its relation to atherosclerosis. *Ann. Rev. Biochem.,* 46:897-930, 1977.

15. Johnson, M.L., B.S. Burke, and J. Mayer. Relative importance of inactivity and overeating in the energy balance of obese high school girls. *Am. J. Clin. Nutr.,* 4(1):36-44, 1956.

16. Khoury, P., J.A. Morrison, K. Kelly, M. Mellies, R. Horvitz, and C.J. Glueck. Clustering and interrelationships of coronary heart disease risk factors in schoolchildren, ages 6-19. *Am. J. Epid.,* 112(4):524-538, 1980.

17. Kobayashi, K., K. Kitamura, and M. Muira. Aerobic power as related to body growth and training in Japanese boys: A longitudinal study. *J. Appl. Physiol.,* 44:666-672, 1978.

18. Kramsch, D.M., A.J. Aspen, B.M. Abramowitz, T. Kremendahl, and W.B. Hood. Reduction of coronary atherosclerosis by moderate conditioning exercise in monkeys on an atherogenic diet. *N.E.J. Med.,* 305:1483-1489, 1981.

19. Laskarzewski, P., J.A. Morrison, I. deGrott, K.A. Kelly, M.J. Mellies, P. Khoury, and C.J. Glueck. Lipid and lipoprotein tracking in 108 children over a four-year period. *Pediatrics,* 64(5):584-591, 1979.

20. Lauer, R.M., W.E. Connor, P.E. Leaverton, M.A. Reiter, and W.R. Clarke. Coronary heart disease risk factors in school children: The Muscatine study. *J. Pediatr.,* 86(5):697-706, 1975.

21. MacConnie, S.E., T.B. Gilliam, D.L. Geenen, and A.E. Pels. Daily physical activity patterns of prepubertal children involved in a rigorous exercise program. *Int. J. Sports Med.,* 3(4):202-207, 1982.

22. McGill, H.C., J.C. Geer, and J.P. Strong. "Natural history of human atherosclerotic lesions." In *Atherosclerosis and its origins,* edited by M. Sandler and G.H. Bourne, pp. 39-66. New York: Academic Press, 1963.

23. McNamara, J., M.A. Malot, J.F. Stremple, and R.R. Cutting. Coronary artery disease in combat casualties in Viet Nam. *JAMA,* 216(7):1185-1187, 1971.

24. Marmot, M.G. Epidemiological basis for the prevention of coronary heart disease. *WHO,* 57(3):331-347, 1979.

25. Pearson, T.A., J.M. Dillman, K. Solex, and R.H. Heptistall. Evidence for two populations of fatty streaks with different roles in the atherogenic process. *Lancet,* 2(8193):496-498, 1980.

26. Pooling Project Research Group. Relationship of blood pressure, serum cholesterol, smoking habit, relative weight and ECG abnormalities to incidence of major coronary events: Final report of the Pooling Project. *J. Chron. Dis.,* 31:201-306, 1978.

27. Rose, H.E., and J. Mayer. Activity, calories intake, fat storage and energy balance of infants. *Pediatrics,* 41(1):18-29, 1959.

28. Ross, R., and L. Harker. Heperlipidemia and atherosclerosis. *Science,* 193:1094-1100, 1976.

29. Saris, W.M.H., R.A. Binkhurst, A.B. Cramwinckel, F. Waesberghe, and A.M. Veen-Hezemans. "The relationship between working performance, daily physical activity, fatness, blood lipids and nutrition in school children." In *Children and exercise IX,* edited by K. Berg and B.O. Ericksson, pp. 166-174. Baltimore: University Park Press, 1980.

30. Savage, P.J., R.F. Hamman, G. Bartha, S.E. Dippe, M. Miller, and P.H. Bennet. Serum cholesterol levels in American (Pima) Indian children and adolescents. *Pediatrics,* 58(2):274-282, 1976.

31. Seliger, V., Z. Trefny, S. Bartunkova, and M. Pauer. The habitual activity and physical fitness of twelve-year-old boys. *Acta. Paediatr. Belg.,* 28:54-59, 1974.

32. Strong, J.P., and H.C. McGill. The pediatric aspects of atherosclerosis. *J. Atheroscl. Res.,* 9:251-265, 1969.

33. Strong, J.P., D.A. Eggen, and M.C. Oalmann. "The natural history, geographic pathology and epidemiology of atherosclerosis." In *The pathogenesis of atherosclerosis,* edited by R.W. Wissler and J.C. Geer, pp. 20-40. Baltimore: Williams & Wilkins, 1972.

34. Taskinen, M.R., and E.A. Nikkila. Lipoprotein lipase of adipose tissue and skeletal muscle in human obesity: Response to glucose and semistarvation. *Metabolism,* 30(8):810-817, 1981.

35. Terjung, R.L. "Endocrine response to exercise." In *Exercise and sport sciences reviews* (Vol. 7), edited by R.S. Hutton and D.I. Miller, pp. 153-180. Philadelphia: Franklin Institute, 1979.

36. Waxman, M., and A.J. Stunkard. Caloric intake and energy expenditure of obese boys. *J. Pediatr.,* 96(2):187-193, 1980.

37. Weninger, M., K. Widhalm, W. Strobl, and G. Schernthaner. Childhood obesity: Serum lipoproteins, glucose and insulin concentrations after an oral glucose load. *Artery,* 8(2):185-190, 1980.

38. Wilmore, J.H., and J.J. McNamara. Prevalence of coronary disease risk factors in boys, 8 to 12 years of age. *J. Pediatr.,* 84:527-533, 1974.

39. Wissler, R.W. Development of the atherosclerotic plaque. In *The myocardium: Failure and infarction*, edited by E. Braunwald, pp. 155-175. New York: H.P. Publishing, 1974.

40. Velican, D., and C. Velican. Study of fibrous plaques occurring in coronary arteries of children. *Atheroscl.,* 33:201-215, 1979.

41. Velican, D., and C. Velican. Atherosclerotic involvement of the coronary arteries of adolescents and young adults. *Atheroscl.,* 36:449-460, 1980.

42. Voller, R.D., and W.B. Strong. Pediatric aspects of atherosclerosis. *Am. Heart J.,* 101(6):815-836, 1981.

9

Overuse Syndromes of the Lower Extremity in Youth Sports

Jack T. Andrish
Cleveland Clinic Foundation

The majority of sports injuries in children involve management of overuse syndromes. The Section of Sports Medicine at the Cleveland Clinic evaluates over 2,000 new injuries a year. Of these, 20% occur in individuals age 15 and under. In this population, over 40% of the new injuries that we see are directly related to overuse of the affected parts. Some 72% of these injuries will affect the lower extremities, 19% the upper extremities, and 9% the spine. The literature has suggested to some extent that overuse syndromes in children are directly related to the level of organization in their sport (10,12,25,26,39,44). That is, overuse syndromes in the child who participates only in neighborhood athletics are uncommon. However, as one becomes more organized and "dedicated" to achievement in a particular sport, the incidence of overuse syndromes rises. This presentation will be confined to the diagnosis and management of various physical syndromes that are encountered in a sports medicine practice involving children. The philosophical aspects of overuse and abuse have been dealt with by others.

As already mentioned, approximately 72% of childhood injuries that are seen in our sports medicine clinic are related to the lower extremity. Of these injuries to the lower extremity, 64% involve the knee, 11% involve the ankle, and 8% directly involve the foot. The remainder of lower extremity problems are distributed among the hip, thigh, and lower leg regions.

INJURIES TO THE LOWER EXTREMITY

Foot

Although the foot would seem to be a frequent victim of overuse in children, it appears to be remarkably resistant to injury. While stress syndromes of tendons and bone do occur, they are rarely associated with long-term disability.

Severe's Disease. Endochondral ossification is our primary means of longitudinal growth mediated through the growth plates (physes) of long bones. However, there are cartilagenous growth plates about the body that contribute more to form and conture of bone rather than to longitudinal growth. These apophyses further serve as sites of insertion or origin of muscle-tendon units. A common example is the posterior calcaneal apophysis. The tendo-Achilles inserts into this area of the calcaneous and may at times become a source of tenderness and pain. The pain is located about the heel and may be either directly at the site of insertion of the Achilles tendon within the calcaneous or, most commonly, directly beneath the heel. The pain is aggravated by contact during heel strike in walking or running. It may be aggravated by push off, as in sprinting or jumping, and it is relieved by rest. X-rays obtained of the heel demonstrate an apparent sclerosis and fragmentation of the calcaneal apophysis. The radiographic findings are really variations of normal and the diagnosis itself is strictly a clinical one. The syndrome is felt to represent a chronic traction strain on the apophysis with resulting micro-trauma and inflammation.

It usually occurs in active preadolescents and is best managed by the insertion of a heel pad for shock absorption at heel strike and Achilles tendon stretching exercises to improve overall flexibility of the muscle-tendon unit (36). Activities that aggravate pain may have to be temporarily curtailed if a heel pad alone does not afford relief. It has not been necessary in our practice to immobilize children with Severe's disease in short leg casts, although a "resistant" case may benefit from this treatment. Invasive management such as through cortisone (or steroid) injections have no place in this condition. At its very worst, it is a benign, self-limiting condition.

Pes Planus. The flexible flat foot is a common occurrence in life but is not usually painful in children (4). However, we have not found an excessive number of children with flexible flat feet and overuse type pain in the lower extremities. If one does come to our clinic with foot pain and is engaged in excessive running and jumping activities, we search for underlying pathology such as stress fracture, structural bone abnormalities, or tarsal coalitions. If the pes planus is flexible and not associated with an underlying disease or congenital bone abnormalities, management with orthotics to prevent excessive pronation can be helpful in reducing strain across this area.

Stress Fracture. Bones are a rather plastic material. They are constantly subjected to bending moments during weightbearing. Repetitive stress can indeed fatigue bone to the point of failure (30). This may happen just as well in the immature skeleton as the mature bone (14,21,41,43). In the foot, the metatarsals are most commonly involved although any bone may be affected. We have seen stress fractures of the tarsal navicular bone as well as the calcaneous in skeletally immature individuals. Any unexplained pain in the foot with localized tenderness over the affected bone should be highly suspect as a stress fracture. Of course, this is providing that the individual has been participating in an activity that involves repetitive running or jumping. Initial x-rays may be entirely normal as stress fractures are usually nondisplaced. It may take approximately 2 to 3 weeks for radiographic changes to occur that more clearly define the location and nature of the stress fracture.

Stress fractures of the calcaneous and metatarsals usually heal quite uneventfully with restriction of running for 3 to 6 weeks. Depending upon the level of pain, a short leg walking cast may or may not be required. The stress fracture of the tarsal navicular does not carry such a benign natural history (38). It may be quite resistant to closed treatment and plaster immobilization, and at times has required operations such as bone grafting or electrical stimulation to encourage proper healing. When plain x-rays are insufficient, bone scans and tomograms have been useful in helping to further diagnose these conditions (Figure 9-1).

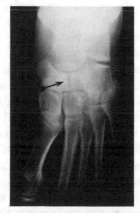

Figure 9-1. Stress fracture of the tarsal navicular can be an elusive diagnosis which may require a bone scan and tomograms to confirm.

Leg

Whereas tendons, ligaments, and bones characterize the anatomy of the foot, muscles and bone predominate in the lower leg. Repetitive microtrauma to the musculature of the leg can lead to various syndromes. The clinical challenge is in establishing a proper and specific diagnosis. Accurate assessment is mandatory since morbidity, disability, and treatment options can be quite diverse.

Shin Splints. The term *shin splints* refers to the syndrome of transient pain in the leg from running or hiking and should exclude stress fractures or ischemic disorders (1). Typically this pain is located over the posterior medial border of the tibia corresponding to various muscle group attachments. True shin splints probably represent a chronic periostitis or inflammation of the fibrous layer covering the bone (13,18). Repetitive microtrauma at the bony origin of muscles in the lower leg produces a chronic benign inflammatory response, which is manifested typically as pain and tenderness (8). The pain, of course, is aggravated by activities such as running and relieved by rest. The diagnosis is really one of exclusion. Proper history taking, x-rays, and at times special diagnostic techniques such as bone scans and intracompartmental pressure monitoring are required to exclude sister diagnoses such as compartment syndromes and stress fracture.

A wealth of mystique and witchcraft surrounds the treatment of shin splints. There have been rational efforts to sort out efficacy of various treatments. When all is said and done, the conclusions suggest that shin splints are typically a benign, self-limiting disorder that uniformly respond to cessation of running (2). Popular treatment modalities that include the use of heel pads, heelcord stretching exercises, nonsteroidal anti-inflammatory medications, and cast immobilization have not been shown to hold a statistically significant advantage over rest alone. There is some evidence, however, that prevention of shin splints is aided by a proper and graduated conditioning program.

Our approach in managing a child with the shin splint syndrome, then, is to first rule out other causes of lower leg pain and then to critically evaluate the amount of activities being performed. An initial period of rest followed by an adjustment in the training routine that allows for a graduated return usually suffices. Frequently, "rest" is merely reducing the amount of running to a level that can be performed comfortably. Typically this is one-half the usual training distance. We would then have the young athlete perform at this level for a week or two and proceed systematically to increase the distance, but at a slow pace. When the desired distance can be completed at a slow pace comfortably, a gradual increase in pace is allowed. Of course, there is some variation in the time that it takes for one to proceed through this shin splint rehabilitation.

Compartment Syndromes. Not all repetitive lower leg pain caused by running is true shin splints. The individual who is quite refractory to the sort of management that we have outlined under shin splints may be considered as having a compartment syndrome (19,29,32,33,37). The muscle groups located in the lower leg are divided into four compartments: anterior, peroneal, superficial, and deep posterior compartments. Muscles included in these compartments are surrounded by a fairly nonyielding outer fascial covering. At times individuals may experience sufficient rise in the intracompartmental pressures during exercise that can result in local ischemia (5,20,23,40). The swelling, ischemia, and local tissue acidosis produce pain and tenderness. Typically this pain comes with activities such as running or sometimes walking, is confined to a particular compartment in the leg, and is relieved by rest.

Compartmental pressures are easily measured by one of several standard techniques. These techniques involve the introduction of a needle into the compartment, with pressures measured and expressed in millimeters of mercury. Pressures of greater than 40 mm of mercury or greater than two-thirds of diastolic blood pressure are usually considered indicative of a compartment syndrome.

The treatment of compartment syndromes, whether acute or chronic, is a surgical one. However, the acute compartment syndrome typically is the result of severe trauma and is a true surgical emergency (24). The treatment of a chronic, intermittent compartment syndrome is somewhat more elective. Both include fasciotomy or release of the overlying fascial compartmental covering.

Knee

As in adults, the school-age athlete also sustains injuries to the knee joint more frequently than any other region of the body. Although the knee at first appears to be a rather simple hinged joint, upon further study one can appreciate the incredible complexity involved in the biomechanics of knee motion. Not only are large stresses propagated about the knee, but a complex obligatory interplay of rotation, gliding, and translation occur between the tibia and femur with normal flexion and extension movements. The knee is highly dependent upon the soft tissues to maintain its anatomic stability and biomechanical integrity.

Chondromalacia of the Patella (Patellofemoral Pain Syndrome). Thirty-seven percent of young people age 15 and under with knee problems come to our clinic with pain localized around the front of the knee and the kneecap; the pain is made worse by activities such as running and is relieved by rest. This symptom complex is very similar to the type of pain that adults experience which often is associated with articular cartilage damage on the patellar surface (17). The chondromalacia of adults, however, is frequently absent or minimal in children presenting with parapatellar knee pain. The label of chondromalacia is frequently applied to young people, but Goodfellow's term of patellofemoral pain syndrome is perhaps more appropriate (16). Some 30% of these young individuals will have lower limb malalignment: they walk and run with their feet straight ahead but their knees tend to be directed inward. This is most noticeable with walking and jogging. The undersurface of the patella is shaped somewhat like the keel on a boat and travels within a groove between the femoral condyles. Abnormalities of this tracking mechanism are frequently associated with patellofemoral pain syndrome. Indeed, full-fledged chondromalacia surface changes beneath the patella can be directly attributed to abnormalities of tracking. The changes that occur in the articular cartilage consist of softening, blistering, and fissuring. Advanced disease can lead to frank cartilage erosions.

Most often, this patellofemoral pain syndrome is a product of overuse. Treatment then is heavily directed toward trying to find the underlying precipitating activities and then modifying them somewhat. Activities that involve deep knee bends, squatting, kneeling, running stairs and so forth are frequent aggravators of this parapatellar pain. Avoiding these activities is often all that is needed.

The patellofemoral pain syndrome includes a spectrum of disease. The mild and early form can be managed simply by modification of activity alone, perhaps as little as a few days of rest. However, persistent symptoms may require more specific treatment.

For good reason a mainstay in the active treatment of chondromalacia traditionally is a physical therapy program that emphasizes quadriceps rehabilitation (11). Specifically, activities to increase the strength of the vastus medialis obliqus have been emphasized in an effort to prevent the lateral subluxation and malalignment of the patella within its femoral groove relationship. Isometric progressive resistance exercises and short arc isotonic progressive resistance exercises have been prescribed to further accomplish this purpose (Figure 9-2). Traditional full arc isotonic progressive resistance exercises usually aggravate the pain and are contraindicated in this condition. As with any exercise rehabilitation program, balance of musculature is as important as ultimate strength and, therefore, hamstring progressive resistance exercises as well as hip flexor and extensor and dorsiflexors and plantar flexor exercises for the ankle are also prescribed. Furthermore, there is evidence especially in young people that tightness of muscle groups about the knee further contribute to this symptom complex (31). Therefore, quadriceps, hamstring, and heelcord stretching exercises are further encouraged.

Braces may be prescribed for symptomatic relief of pain and a whole host of commercial devices are available. One of the simplest and most reliable is the Bike cartilage brace. The spectrum of braces, however, may proceed from the recently proposed patellar strap to the formal

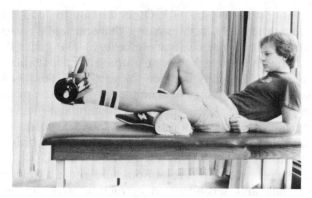

Figure 9-2. With the knee initially flexed to 30 degrees, the patient is asked to straighten the knee and hold for 6 seconds. Three sets of 10 are performed daily, increasing the amount of weight by 2½ lb. increments as tolerated.

patellar stabilization brace of Palumbo (28) as shown in Figure 9-3.

There is no specific medication for the treatment of chondromalacia. However, nonsteroidal anti-inflammatory medications may be beneficial and in particular salicylates may be prescribed on a regular basis, especially if an effusion is present within the joint. It has been suggested that salicylates may further act by primarily affecting the articular cartilage in preventing chondrocyte degradation (6).

More than 90% of young people with parapatellar pain syndromes can be managed effectively and nonoperatively. However, some will be resistant to this form of treatment and will require surgical intervention. Presently this consists of an arthroscopic evaluation to more specifically define the diagnosis, and most treatments commonly proceed with a lateral retinacular release (22). Releasing the lateral retinaculum to some degree improves the tracking mechanism of the patella within the femoral groove and relieves excessive lateral pressure. It appears to be most effective for the individual with parapatellar pain not associated with severe articular cartilage damage or recurrent patellar dislocations.

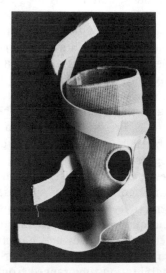

Figure 9-3. The Palumbo brace has been found a useful adjunct in the management of patellofemoral pain syndrome and patellar instability.

Osgood-Schlatter's Disease. In 1903, Osgood of Boston and Schlatter of Zurich independently described an entity characterized by swelling and tenderness of the tibial tubercle in adolescents (27,34). Since that time a great deal of misconception has been propagated about this condition (9). The individual is usually between the ages of 12 and 14 and complains of knee pain. There may be a noticeable nobbiness or bump over the anterior aspect of the knee around the tibial tubercle and this can be exquisitely tender. X-rays demonstrate this area to be an apophyseal growth plate, and characteristically these x-rays may show this apophysis to be fragmented.

The feeling has been that this condition represents an inflammation of the growth plate area secondary to a traction stress applied by the patellar tendon. Biopsies have shown, however, that this actually represents a chronic patellar tendinitis where the patellar tendon inserts into the apophysis. Repeated microtrauma at this tendon insertion sets up an inflammatory response with secondary swelling, pain, and tenderness. It should be remembered and emphasized to the patient and parents that Osgood-Schlatter's disease is a benign, self-limiting condition. Left on its own without treatment, Osgood-Schlatter's disease will resolve itself and will not lead to a damaged or weak knee joint. Only on occasion is the "victim" of Osgood-Schlatter's disease left with a tender calcium deposit within the patellar tendon in later years. Our treatment, then, should not be worse than the disease.

Just as chondromalacia has a spectrum of symptom severities, so does Osgood-Schlatter's disease. Treatment is directed toward symptomatic relief of pain; if the young person has pain only at the beginning or end of sporting activities, and if the pain is of no functional importance, the treatment is essentially observation. Protective knee pads to avoid repeated contusions to the area are probably all that is needed. After the activities, local swelling and tenderness may be controlled with ice. However, if the pain interferes with running activities or if the pain increases the treatment should be more active. Initially, an exercise program is prescribed which emphasizes flexibility including quadricep, hamstring, and heelcord stretching exercises. To some extent the program advised by Henning is carried out by prescribing hamstring strengthening exercises (31). In Henning's study, young people affected with Osgood-Schlatter's disease characteristically demonstrated relative overactivity of their quadriceps musculature and increased tightness of their quadriceps. A program of quadriceps, hamstring, and heelcord stretching exercises and hamstring strengthening exercises relieved the symptoms of Osgood-Schlatter's disease in more than 85% of cases. The rehabilitation time ranged from 3 weeks to 3 months.

There is no specific medication for Osgood-Schlatter's disease, but as with chondromalacia, nonsteroidal anti-inflammatory agents or slicylates may help if swelling and tenderness are excessive. Further, the host of cartilage braces, counterforce braces, and patellar stabilization braces have also been applied to the patient with Osgood-Schlatter's disease with variable effectiveness. Usually elastic knee pads work best by minimizing local trauma to the area. Cortisone injections, advocated by some, are not advocated by this author because of their adverse effects on local tissue. Surgery in the actively growing adolescent is also not recommended. The occasional young adult with the painful ossicle remnant within the patellar tendon, however, can be relieved of symptoms by exercising this calcium deposit.

Jumper's Knee. Perhaps a more resistant problem to treat is the so-called jumper's knee lesion (3). This individual describes generalized anterior knee pain but localized tenderness over the inferior pole of the patella. The pain is aggravated by activities, especially those involving jumping, and is relieved by rest. Recently labeled jumper's knee, this condition actually represents a chronic patellar tendinitis at the patella tendon's origin from the inferior pole of the patella. Again, repeated microtrauma sets up the sequence of chronic benign inflammatory response. However, this sometimes leads to local tissue necrosis within the patellar tendon and reported cystic changes. Ectopic calcification may also be seen adjacent to the inferior pole of the patella at the proximal patellar tendon.

This condition has a greater likelihood of becoming chronic than Osgood-Schlatter's disease and is functionally more incapacitating. It is more resistant to treatment since simple padding of the area affords no relief. For the most part, the advice of Blazina et al. (3) in staging jumper's knee patients and adjusting their treatment appropriately is followed. The overall success rate of exercise, braces, medicines, and even surgery are less effective than it is for Osgood-Schlatter's disease. Patellar tendon ruptures have been reported with chronic jumper's knee patients but these are usually associated with cortisone injections. Treatment consists of generous applications of ice after activity, and exercises that emphasize flexibility. Numerous counterforce braces have been devised and approximately half of these will afford some symptomatic, if incomplete, relief. The very resistant individual who has tolerated at least 3 months of rest and rehabilitation, and yet continues to be symptomatic, may require surgical exploration. The area is debrided of the chronic inflammatory tissue, and the success rate is approximately 50-80%.

Hip

The hip joint is characterized anatomically by great stability. Further, large muscle mass completely comprise the pelvic girdle. The presence of large muscles and inherently stable joints make this region of the body resistant to serious injury. However, repetitive overuse and microtrauma delivered to muscles and their bony origins can result in painful symptom complexes. For the most part these conditions are easily treated and do not produce long-term disability.

Apophysitis. There are numerous apophyses about the hip and pelvic area that serve as sites of origin and insertion for various muscle tendon units. As with Osgood-Schlatter's disease, chronic repeated microtrauma that usually occurs in young people involved in excessive running sports can present as pain around the hip region (15,35). Clancy has best described these various apophyseal injuries to the pelvis and hip region in young runners (7). X-rays sometimes demonstrate partial separation of these growth plate areas resulting from chronic repeated traction type microtrauma.

Treatment centers around a period of rest and then gradual return to activity within the limits of tolerable pain. Permanent sequellae are extremely uncommon except for the avulsed ischial apophysis. The ischium serves as a site of origin of the hamstring muscles and avulsion of this apophysis is usually the result of an acute injury. However, abuse of the symptomatic painful tender ischial apophysis can lead to heterotopic bone formation and disability (Figure 9-4). In fact, surgical excision of these ectopic calcium deposits may be required. The iliac crest, which serves as the site of origin of the abdominal musculature as well as iliolumbar musculature and gluteal musculature, can be involved. The anterior superior iliac spine as well as the anterior inferior iliac spine are frequent offenders as well.

Tendinitis. Most commonly, tendinitis involves the iliotibial band. The iliotibial band originates from the iliac crest and travels distally in conjunction with the tensor fascia latae muscle and eventually terminates at an insertion distal to the knee. This band, however, crosses the greater trochanter of the hip and is separated normally by a bursa. Overuse or

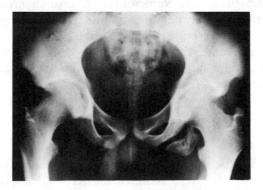

Figure 9-4. This large, painful heterotopic bone formed as a result of an avulsed ischial apophysis. Surgical excision was required.

trauma can result in inflammation of this bursa beneath the iliotibial band. Flexion and extension, especially accompanied by internal rotation, may produce excessive snapping of this iliotibial band over the greater trochanter with subsequent irritation, inflammation, and resulting pain and tenderness. Often the patient will mistakenly believe that his/her hip is dislocating as this iliotibial band snaps over the greater trochanter.

Treatment begins with the reassurance that this is a snapping tendon and not an unstable hip, and proceeds with the usual modalities for the treatment of tendinitis (i.e., rest, ice, rehabilitation exercises, flexibility, and then a gradual return to activity within the limits of pain). Nonsteroidal anti-inflammatory medication may be of benefit here with local ice compresses.

CONCLUSION

The skeletally immature body is to a large extent more forgiving than the skeletally mature one (42). However, overuse and abuse can certainly occur in a young person. The syndromes and symptom complexes resulting from overuse can result in breakdown of tissue and secondary inflammatory responses. The young body has a great capacity for tissue repair and remodeling. The basic underlying treatment of any overuse syndrome in the young growing person is a period of rest that allows the body's natural repair mechanisms to take over. This repair is usually *complete*; long-term adaptive and compensatory adjustments, whether in the form of orthotics, techniques, or surgeries, are usually not indicated as they frequently are in the older individual. However, there are natural limits even in a child, and exceeding these limits can lead to needless permanent damage.

REFERENCES

1. American Medical Association. *Subcommittee on classification of sports injuries: Standard nomenclature of athletic injuries,* pp. 122-216. Chicago: American Medical Association, 1966.

2. Andrish, J.T., J.A. Bergfeld, and J. Walheim. A prospective study of the management of shin splints. *J. Bone & Joint Surg.,* 56A(8):1697-1700, 1974.

3. Blazina, M.E., R.K. Kerlan, F.W. Jobe, V.S. Carter, and G.J. Carlson. Jumper's knee. *Orthopedic Clin. of N. Amer.,* 4(3):665-678, 1973.

4. Bleck, E.E., and U.J. Berzins. Conservative management of pes valgus with plantar flexed talus, flexible. *Clin. Ortho. & Rel. Res.,* 122:85-94, 1977.

5. Brooker, A.F., and C. Pezeshki. Tissue pressure to evaluate compartmental syndrome. *J. Trauma,* 19(9):689-691, 1979.

6. Chrisman, O.D., and G.A. Snook. Studies in the protective effect of aspirin against degeneration of human articular cartilage. *Clin. Orthopedics,* 56:77, 1968.

7. Clancy, W.G., and A.S. Foltz. Iliac apophysitis and stress fractures in adolescent runners. *Amer. J. Sports Med.,* 4(5):214-218, 1976.

8. Clement, D.B. Tibial stress syndrome in athletes. *J. of Sports Med.,* 2(2):81-85, 1974.

9. D'Ambrosia, R.D., and G.L. MacDonald. Pitfalls in the diagnosis of Osgood-Schlatter's disease. *Clin. Ortho. & Rel. Res.,* 110:206-209, 1975.

10. DeHaven, K.E. Athletic injuries in adolescents. *Pediatric Ann.,* 7(10):96-119, 1978.

11. DeHaven, E.K., W.A. Dolan, and P.J. Mayer. Chondromalacia patella in athletes—Clinical presentation and conservative management. *Amer. J. Sports Med.,* 7:1-12, 1979.

12. DeHaven, K.E., and C.M. Evarts. Throwing injuries of the elbow in athletes. *Ortho. Clin. of N. Amer.,* 4(3):801-808, 1973.

13. Devas, M.B., and R. Sweetnam. Stress fractures of the tibia in athletes or "shin soreness." *J. Bone & Joint Surg.,* 4:227-239, 1958.

14. Engh, C.A., R.A. Robinson, and J. Milgram. Stress fractures in children. *J. Trauma,* 10(7):532-541, 1970.

15. Godshall, R.W., and C.A. Hansen. Incomplete avulsion of a portion of the iliac epiphysis. An injury of young athletes. *J. Bone & Joint Surg.,* 55A(6):1301-1302, 1973.

16. Goodfellow, J., D.S. Hungerford, and C. Woods. Patellofemoral joint mechanics and pathology. Chondromalacia Patellae. *J. Bone & Joint Surg.,* 58B(3):291-299, 1976.

17. Johnson, P.H. Chondromalacia patellae. *J. Ark. Med. Soc.,* 76(3):142-147, August 1979.

18. LaCave, G. Enthesis—Traumatic disease of insertions. *J. Amer. Med. Assoc.,* 169:254-255, 1959.

19. Leach, R.E., G. Hammond, and W.S. Stryker. Anterior tibial compartment syndrome—Active and chronic. *J. Bone & Joint Surg.,* 49A(3):451-462, 1967.

20. Matsen, F.A., K.A. Mayo, G.W. Sheridan, and R.B. Krugmire. Monitoring of intramuscular pressure. *Surgery,* 79(6):702-709, 1976.

21. McBryde, A.M. Stress fractures in athletes. *J. Sports Med.,* 3(5):212-217, 1975.

22. Micheli, L.J., and C.L. Stanitski. Lateral patellar retinacular release. *Amer. J. Sports Med.,* 9(5):330-336, 1981.

23. Mubarak, S.J., A.R. Hargens, C.A. Owen, L.P. Garetto, and W.H. Akeson. The Wick Catheter technique for measurement of in-

tramuscular pressure. A new research and clinic tool. *J. Bone & Joint Surg.*, 58A:1016-1020, 1976.

24. Mubarak, S.J., C.A. Owen, A.R. Hargens, L.P. Garetto, and W.H. Akeson. Compartment syndromes. Diagnosis and treatment with the aid of the wick catheter. *J. Bone & Joint Surg.*, 60A(8):1091-1095, 1978.

25. Orava, S., and J. Puranen. Exertion injuries of adolescent athletes. *Brit. J. Sports Med.*, 12:4-10, 1978.

26. Orava, S., and J. Saarela. Exertion injuries to young athletes. A follow-up research of orthopedic problems of young track and field athletes. *Amer. Sports Med.*, 6(2):68-74, 1978.

27. Osgood, R.B. Lesions of the tibial tubercle occurring during adolescence. *Boston Med. Surg. J.*, 148:114, 1903.

28. Palumbo, P.M. Dynamic patellar brace: A new orthosis in the management of patellofemoral disorders. A preliminary report. *Amer. J. Sports Med.*, 9(1):45-49, 1981.

29. Paul, W.D., and G.L. Soderberg. "The shin splint confusion." In *Proceedings of eighth national conference on the medical aspects of sports*, pp. 19-23. Chicago, American Medical Association.

30. Pentecost, R.L., R.A. Murray, and H.H. Brindley. Fatigue, insufficiency, and pathologic fractures. *J. Amer. Med. Assoc.*, 187(13):1001-1004, 1964.

31. Personal communication with Charles Henning, M.D., Wichita, Kansas.

32. Puranen, J. The medial tibial syndrome. Exercise ischemia in the medial fascial compartment of the leg. *J. Bone & Joint Surg.*, 56B(4):712-715, 1974.

33. Reneman, R.S. The anterior and the lateral compartmental syndrome of the leg due to intensive use of muscles. *Clin. Ortho. & Rel. Res.*, 113:69-80, 1975.

34. Schlatter, C. Verletzugen des Schnabelformigen Fortsatzes der Oberen Tibiaepiphyse. *Beritz Z Klin Chir Tubing*, 38:874-887, 1903.

35. Schlonsky, J., and M.l. Olix. Functional disability following avulsion of the ischial epiphysis. Report of two cases. *J. Bone & Joint Surg.*, 54A(3):641-644, 1972.

36. Seder, J.I. Heel injuries incurred in running and jumping. *Physician & Sportsmed.*, 4(10):70-73, 1976.

37. Slocum, D.B. "The shin splints syndrome. Medical aspects and differential diagnosis." In *Proceedings of eighth national conference on the medical aspects of sports*, pp. 24-31. Chicago, American Medical Association.

38. Torg, J.S., H. Pavlov, L.H. Cooley, M.H. Bryant, S.P. Arnoczky, J.A. Bergfeld, and L.Y. Hunter. Stress fractures of the tarsal navicular. *J. Bone & Joint Surg.*, 64A(5):700-712, 1982.

39. Torg, J.S., H. Pollack, and P. Sweterlitsch. Effect of competitive pitching on the shoulders and elbows of preadolescent baseball players. *Pediatrics*, 49(2):267-271, 1972.

40. Walter, N.E., & M.D. Wolf. Stress fractures in young athletes. *Amer. J. Sports Med.,* 5(4):165-170, 1979.

41. Whitesides, T.E., T.C. Haney, K. Marimoto, and H. Harada. Tissue pressure measurements as a determinant for the need of fasciotomy. *Clin. Ortho. & Rel. Res.,* 113:43-51, 1975.

42. Wilkens, K.E. The uniqueness of the young athlete: musculo-skeletal injuries. *Amer. J. Sports Med.,* 8(5):377-382, 1980.

43. Wilson, E.S., and F.N. Katz. Stress fractures—An analysis of 250 consecutive cases. *Radiology*, 92:481-486, 1969.

44. Zaricznyk, B., L.J.M. Shattuck, T.A. Mast, R.V. Robertson, and G. E'Elia. Sports-related injuries in school-aged children. *Amer. J. Sports Med.,* 8(5):318-324, 1980.

Index